THE 100-DAY RECLAIM

THE 100-DAY RECLAIM

DAILY READINGS TO MAKE HEALTH AND FITNESS AS EMPOWERING AS IT SHOULD BE

Nia Shanks

Copyright © by Nia Shanks

All rights reserved. This book or any portion thereof may not be reproduced or used in any manner whatsoever without the express written permission of the author.

www.NiaShanks.com

ISBN: 978-1-69657-714-4

CONTENTS

Disclaimer vi

Preface vii

Introduction 1

Days 1–10 3

Days 11–20 21

Days 21-30 37

Days 31–40 53

Days 41–50 71

Days 51–60 91

Days 61–70 109

Days 71–80 131

Days 81–90 149

Days 91–100 167

Conclusion 183

About the Author 185

DISCLAIMER

This book is for educational and entertainment purposes and should not be used as a substitute for professional medical treatment, advice, or diagnosis. Consult your physician or health-care provider before changing your diet or starting an exercise/strength training program to determine if it is right for your needs.

PREFACE

To not constantly be thinking about food—what you "should" or "shouldn't" eat. Not looking at your body and instantly seeing flaws or features you dislike. Not feeling guilty for skipping a workout or eating your favorite dessert. Not fighting against your body to lose weight or improve your health. Not having your entire day ruined from the number you see on the bathroom scale in the morning.

Enjoying the process of working out, instead of dreading it. Eating with enjoyment, rather than guilt, shame, or deprivation. Appreciating your body in new, empowering ways. Building a health and fitness lifestyle that enhances and improves your life, instead of dominating it.

It's not fiction. It's not a fantasy. It can be your reality.

Health and fitness has been contorted. Mangled. In its current state, it's not about making us better versions of ourselves, or even *healthier* versions. The way popular trends would have it, food must be earned, our bodies must fit a certain mold, and exercise is punishment for "blowing your diet." Diets are defined by deprivation and must-avoid foods, while workout programs glamorize soreness and exhaustion. All this is causing women to be dissatisfied with their bodies, to have a bad relationship with food, and to dread anything involving fitness because of the negative connotation attached to it.

But no more. It's time to reclaim health and fitness and make it a lifestyle that works for you. Something that builds you up. Something that is simple and sustainable, enjoyable and empowering. To complement, not dominate, your life.

This book will show you the way, with daily readings and lessons you will practice over the next one hundred days. Commit to this journey, do your part each day, and you'll be rewarded not just when you reach the end, but each step of the way.

INTRODUCTION

This book has a singular purpose: To help you simplify health and fitness so you can achieve your goals in an enjoyable, empowering, sustainable fashion and divorce from food and fitness all the unnecessary frustration, morality, judgment, and stress that has become enmeshed with it.

But for that to happen, dear reader, you must do your part.

It's not enough to simply read each daily passage, then forget about this book until the following day when it's time to read the next entry. You must *practice* what you read. You must put each lesson to use, each and every day, for the next one hundred days.

In the same way you can't simply read through a workout program and reap results from it, or read about simple nutrition changes and improve your health without actually practicing them, neither can you experience results from reading a passage in this book and instantly forgetting about it until you read the next one tomorrow.

You must apply the information. Daily.

How to be successful with this book: Read a passage in the morning, keep its lesson in mind as you go throughout the day, actively practice the lesson when applicable, then review how you did in the evening. It may help to reread the day's passage as you ruminate over your practice.

Journaling can also be useful. As you read each lesson, write down the thoughts that are prompted, along with how you did and what you learned throughout the day as you put it into practice. This is a powerful exercise you can do every day for the next one hundred days.

Commit now to not simply reading each daily passage, then going about business as usual. Read each entry, digest it, apply its lessons as best you can. Then review your application of it in the evening. If you're willing to record your thoughts and experiences in a daily journal, even better.

Let's begin.

Days 1–10

Day 1
CHANGE YOUR FOCUS.

If you're like many women, you've gone through a period of years, or even decades, when you focused on losing weight and looking "better." The reasons for working out and eating well were solely for changing the way your body looked in (and out of) clothes. To make the number on the scale go down, or to ensure it didn't creep up. To shrink your waist. To "fix" features about your body you disliked.

"I want to lose weight so I look better." "I want to make sure I don't gain weight so I don't look worse." "I want to fix this flaw." Thoughts like these fuel countless women's food choices and keep them going to the gym week after week.

It's no wonder so many women view health and fitness as a chore. This negativity-fueled focus has only been magnified over the years, thanks to social media and the images flooding our smartphones and computer screens.

Despite living in the twenty-first century, it's difficult for women not to feel that *how we look* is still the most important thing about us. That our body's shape, size, and weight define us.

But you can shift your focus and no longer allow the *I-must-lose-weight* and *I-hate-how-my-body-looks* thoughts fuel your actions.

Stop trying to hate your way to results.

"But if I didn't care about how I look, I'd never go to the gym," you may think. Why then should you work out? To get stronger. To discover what your body *is capable of doing*. To improve your quality of life. To increase your stamina and endurance. To do something that makes you feel great about yourself. Shift the focus from being about *how you look* to *what you can do* (e.g.: run faster or further, lift heavier weights, perform push-ups for the first time). And guess what? It's very possible the results you've desired all along will come as a side effect from the achievement of those empowering goals.

Fitness, strength training, and any activity that gets you moving your body regularly should be an enjoyable, empowering activity that makes you marvel at your body's unique strengths and abilities.

Why do you work out? What thoughts drive your actions, and how can you make them positive, empowering, and enjoyable?

Day 2
THIS IS YOUR JOURNEY.

Don't build sustainable eating habits or enjoyable workout habits to win the praise or admiration of others.

It doesn't matter what you look like now or what you look like one year from now—someone, somewhere, will always find something negative to say about your body.

The solution is to eat well and move your body often for yourself. Treat other people's opinions with indifference. Praise or compliments can be appreciated, but they shouldn't be motivation or validation. Insults or inconsiderate remarks shouldn't concern you, make you question yourself, or dampen your resolve.

You can't control or change what anyone thinks or says about you. Let that truth soak in. Because you have no control over their thoughts or opinions, doesn't it stand to reason that you shouldn't be concerned with them?

What matters is that you do this for yourself. Impress *yourself*.

A snake sheds its skin to allow for growth and to remove parasites. We can become bound up in the opinions expressed by other people (or merely *our expectations* of what we assume other people think) to the point where our growth is stunted. Free yourself from those constraints. Let them fall away so you can continue to grow.

How have the opinions of others affected you? What can you do, today, to help slough away those constraints?

Day 3

THE PROCESS, NOT THE PRIZE.

What is The Prize you seek to attain from your health and fitness efforts? Maybe you want to reach a healthy bodyweight or waist measurement. Maybe you want to be able to play with your children without fatiguing quickly. Maybe you want to win a race or competition. Maybe you want to feel confident in short sleeves. Maybe you want to build muscle.

Lusting after The Prize can be a fatal mistake when it distracts your attention from what ultimately matters: The Process.

What is The Process? The Process consists of the necessary actions, done repeatedly and consistently, that produce (or at least get us closer to) The Prize. Since The Process alone is what produces The Prize, it stands to reason that we should focus our attention and efforts on it.

What *must* you do in order to get close to achieving The Prize you desire? Do not neglect what is right in front of you, the actions demanded of you, because you're trying to look beyond it into the future. What can you do *today* that will take you closer to the goal?

Take advantage of what you have control over—what you choose to do right now, today. What actions can you take this day that will take you closer to The Prize? After all, The Prize won't appear unless you put in the work. It makes sense, then, to focus intently on The Process. To do what must be done *today*, since today is the only thing you have control over.

There is no guarantee you'll attain The Prize you desire. You can do all the workouts, eat all the meals, get sufficient sleep, but still not win the competition. Nothing is for certain, except that nothing you relish achieving comes without putting in the work and embracing The Process.

Today, don't just ask yourself "What are the things I must do to achieve the results I'm after, or to build the lifestyle I want?" Do them.

Day 4
YOU'RE GOING TO MESS UP.

No one wants to stress themselves out unnecessarily, yet that's what we inadvertently do with food and fitness when we try to avoid messing up at all costs.

You can't avoid occasional mess-ups; perfection isn't going to happen. Why do we even expect (or worse, demand) such a preposterous standard in the first place?

Sorry to break it to you, but you're going to miss workouts. At the very least, you'll have to modify them to deal with time constraints, aches or pains, equipment limitations, illness.

And regardless of the nutrition habits you've built, you will overeat. You will eat more than a reasonable serving of dessert or your favorite meal. You will at some point choose the food you crave with all its sugary, fatty, decadent goodness instead of choosing a veggie- and protein-packed salad.

And it's okay!

Don't make unrealistic demands, like never "messing up." All that does is set you up for inevitable failure that will conclude with a hefty amount of frustration.

The solution is simple: Focus on the entirety of your workout and nutrition habits. Don't go for "all or nothing"; go for *often, mostly, regularly, consistently*. Move your body *often* in ways you enjoy. Eat *mostly* minimally-processed, nutrient-dense foods. Do these actions *regularly* and the occasional "mess-up" doesn't mean anything. Really, it's not even a "mess-up"; it's just life.

Take the stigma out of self-declared mess-ups. Laugh them off or, at the very least, accept them, knowing perfection is a myth. Then move on.

Want to put this to practice? Recall a recent self-declared "mess-up" with your fitness or food choices, and view it through this lens.

Day 5
REMOVE THE COLORED GLASSES.

If each morning, before rolling out of bed, you put on a pair of glasses with blue lenses, you'd go about the day viewing everything through a bluish tint. While at first it would seem odd, eventually, as time passed, the blue-tinted world would be normal. You'd forget the blue lenses were artificially coloring everything you saw. To you, the blue tint cast on the world would simply be how the world looked.

The way you view food and fitness can be tinted with the lenses you're wearing. Maybe, instead of color, the lenses you've become accustomed to wearing paint food choices with obsession, anxiety, and guilt. Maybe fitness is distorted with a perception of punishment, a loathsome chore to perform, or a tool to transform a body you don't like seeing in the mirror.

Years of yo-yo dieting, inconsistent fitness habits, life challenges, society, and the information we've ingested have shaped and colored the lens we view these things through, creating a distortion of reality.

This is why two people can stare at the same thing, like a cupcake, but see something entirely different. One person may simply see a tasty dessert; they'll enjoy it, then go about their life without a second thought about the cupcake. The other person may see something "bad" that's loaded with calories that can undo their progress if they eat it, all while calculating in their mind how much exercise they must perform to "burn it off" should they choose to eat it, and then they'll be ravaged with guilt if they do.

Once you realize you're seeing events and habits through colored lenses, you can choose to remove them. By first becoming aware of the lens that's currently distorting your perception, you'll remove a lot of its power.

Think about how you currently view working out and eating healthfully. Has your vision become distorted? In what ways? How can you begin to remove that lens?

Day 6
WHAT DEFINES YOU?

Does the number displayed on the bathroom scale define who you are? Does your clothing size, or your age, the number of pounds lost or gained, or your body shape define *who you are*?

Of course not. But thanks to the rampant nonsense in the health and fitness world, it's difficult not to believe there's some truth to these prevalent fallacies.

The great news, however, is that *you* get to decide what defines you. At every moment. Even this very instant.

What type of person do you want to be? What qualities do you want to define you? Strength, perseverance, kindness, determination, patience, honesty, resilience, humility, courage, dignity? Surely you want the things you do in the world and in your daily life—your actions—to be the traits that define you.

Brush off any implications that your value and self-worth are determined by any arbitrary numbers or shapes or standards.

Examine how you currently tend to determine your self-worth. Then decide what it is you want to define who you are, and the things you will no longer allow to influence you.

Day 7
DAILY ACTIONS.

What if we weren't consumed with the desired outcomes of our actions?

What if, instead, we focused on mastering the skills, principles, and actions that create the healthy lifestyle we want to live? They are, after all, where our energy and time is spent.

Instead of worrying about the number on the scale going down, we get better at eating nourishing meals we enjoy, for their own sake and not just because we want to change the appearance or weight of our bodies.

Instead of obsessing over food or fearing certain foods because of the incorrect labels we've assigned to them—"bad," "dirty," "guilty pleasures"—we commit to removing these labels to eradicate the anxiety we feel around those foods.

Instead of every workout contributing to sculpting muscle or burning fat, we look at each session like a dose of life-promoting medicine.

The actions, done for their own sake, can be enough. Arguably, they should be enough because it's the actions we take over and over, day after day, that define the life we live and determine our well-being.

Small increments of progress should be acknowledged and celebrated. Things like refusing to experience guilt after overindulging, doing a workout despite not "feeling like it," listening to your body and adjusting the workout instead of trying to push through a nagging ache, not partaking of every snack and dessert offered to you and eating instead the ones you enjoy most in a reasonable quantity.

How do you think your week would go, and how would it be different, if you focused on mastering the skills that create the lifestyle you want to live, instead of being blinded by the outcomes they can produce?

Day 8

MANY WINS GO UNACKNOWLEDGED.

With our culture's unrelenting obsession with physical appearance, it's easy to succumb to the suggestion that the only wins that count are the ones that show up on the bathroom scale, body measurements, changes in clothing size, before and after photos.

But there are other wins you should be proud of too:

- Doing a workout, especially when you didn't feel like it.
- Consistently practicing a new habit, like eating a fiber- and protein-rich breakfast.
- Adding more weight to the barbell or hoisting heavier dumbbells.
- Getting out of your comfort zone to try a new exercise, or crushing the intimidation you once felt with certain exercises.
- Managing stress by investing in self-care, such as reading in the evening or going for a leisurely walk.
- Rejecting negative self-talk that creeps into your mind and refusing to give assent to it.
- Seeing food as neither good nor bad, but simply as *food*.
- Refusing to feel guilty after overindulging and getting back to your preferred habits with the next meal.
- Skipping a workout because a great opportunity presented itself and you know that delaying one workout for one day won't set you back in the big picture.

Don't lose sight of these wins. You can collect several in a single day. That is your challenge today: Collect as many wins as you can that have nothing to do with your physical appearance. Pay close attention and you may be surprised at what you discover.

Day 9
THE DANGER OF DEMANDS.

Most women have specific goals they want to achieve from their fitness program. With pinpoint accuracy, they identify where they want to see the greatest improvement: "I want to get rid of my underarm flab." "I need to get rid of this fluff around my midsection." "I want to deadlift twice my bodyweight within the year."

Having a target to aim at is helpful. It guides your actions and ignites motivation. Yet there's a hidden danger to this demand-driven focus. With fat loss, for example, we can't control where the body will shed it first. Our bodies are not stone; we can't chisel away the bits we want to be rid of with meticulous precision. Physiology doesn't work that way.

The danger lies in lusting after an outcome you can't completely control. Demand flab-free upper arms all you want, but you can't control exactly when throughout the process it will happen. When you *demand* a specific result, you're only set up for potential disappointment if it doesn't happen how or when you want it to. Worse, though, you blind yourself from seeing what you *did* accomplish.

The woman who demanded she be able to fit into a size eight within a few months, yet didn't reach that goal, will feel like she failed. Because she didn't attain the exact goal she demanded, she doesn't see all that she did achieve: Her strength increased greatly, she has muscle definition in her legs, her work capacity improved, she built muscle and bone and lost fat, she further ingrained the habit of working out consistently, she gets higher quality sleep, her blood pressure improved.

This long list of positive results goes unnoticed, all because she demanded a specific outcome that hasn't yet been achieved.

You can have *preferences*, but don't make the mistake of

demanding specific outcomes. Put effort into the actions that will take you closer to what you prefer, and savor the results you reap along the journey. Be on the lookout for benefits you didn't even consider, collecting them like little gems you happen to stumble upon, with gratitude.

Think about your journey. What are some benefits you've achieved that you may have overlooked because you were chasing a specific result?

Day 10
WHO WILL YOU BE TODAY?

There's a lot you never had control over, and much more you never will.

You weren't able to select your parents, and thus you can't change your genetic makeup.

You can't control what other people say or think about you.

You can't control the weather and stop it from interfering with your plans.

But you can control how you respond to these things. You control how you choose to use them.

Keep that in mind today with whatever happens. If someone says something hurtful or ignorant, that's a reflection of *them*. You can choose to not let it soak into your skin and affect you.

Likewise, you can choose to make all things related to your health and fitness lifestyle something that makes you better, or breaks you down.

You can build a stronger, healthier body out of desire to collect "likes" and praise on social media that give you fleeting motivation or satisfaction, or you can demand more. You can choose to work out for you, because it makes you feel great about yourself and provides something deeper and more meaningful than the perfect selfie. Perhaps you can also inspire others around you who are looking for a more fulfilling health and fitness journey of their own.

Every day is a new opportunity to choose who you will be.

When things don't go the way you plan today or you face an unexpected challenge, who will you be in response?

Days 11-20

Day 11
JUST STOP DIGGING.

How many times have you eaten a dessert or calorie-rich meal, then rationalized "I already screwed up by eating dessert, so it'll make no difference if I eat whatever I want all weekend and start over on Monday"?

This is something many of us have done. Instead of resuming our regular habits, or getting back to *building* the habits we want to develop, we tell ourselves that we messed up so we might as well keep messing up until we have a nice and neat day to start over again fresh. After all, whoever heard of "getting back on track" on a Saturday evening? The diet restarts Monday.

Not only is this mindset woefully unhelpful, but it's also severely flawed.

If you found yourself stuck in a hole, proceeding to dig it deeper would never be a consideration. Yet that's what we do when we overeat, or miss a workout, or go on a tirade about the features we dislike about our bodies and we feel bad for feeding those old habits we're trying to break, and then feel worse for feeling bad!

We irrationally choose to compound our mistakes. We pick up a shovel and dig at a furious pace, while vowing to stop digging the next day, or Monday, or on New Year's Day. But we could stop digging at any moment. After the first less-than-ideal choice, even after the first several shovel loads, but we often don't.

When you find yourself in a hole, no matter how shallow or deep it is, the response should be the same: Just stop digging.

What is a common situation you find yourself in where you continue to dig the hole deeper? What could you do to ensure you "just stop digging" when you face it again?

Day 12

LEAD WITH YOUR ASS.

Do not underestimate the power of leading with your ass as Mary, a pediatrician, race car driver, and coaching group member explains: "Change doesn't happen in my life by listening to the shit in my head. Change in my life is led by my ass. If my ass goes to the gym and gets it done, my life gets just a teeny bit better. Maybe I won't even notice. But if my ass keeps going, one day I turn around, and my body is strong, and I'm just a little happier."

That message is simple, yet oh-so powerful: Focus on *action*. It can occasionally feel like your brain is working against you rather than helping you achieve your goals, so it may behoove you to put your ass in charge instead.

Here's a common brain-to-ass conversation you can likely relate to that will bring this to life.

Brain: "I don't feel like working out. Let's sit on the couch with a carton of ice cream and dig in with a jumbo-sized serving spoon to achieve maximum ice-cream-to-mouth efficiency."

Ass: "How about letting me take the lead instead, since Brain is clearly not up to the task today? Let's just get to the gym and start the workout. Once you get going, you'll be glad you're there putting in the work. Even if it's not a particularly great workout, you'll feel better once it's done."

Sometimes our brain leads us in the right direction ("I feel amazing! Let's do this!"). Sometimes it's an uncooperative tyrant who would rather dive face first into a kiddie pool filled with fire ants than do something productive.

On days when your brain just isn't cooperating, try putting your ass in charge.

Show up. Do the work. Build momentum through action, no matter how small it may seem.

Day 13

THE NAKED TRUTH, PART I.

Have you ever considered what you're *really* doing when you work out? When you deadlift, for example, you are picking up a symmetrically loaded piece of steel, then putting it back down. Then you pick it up again. You are merely lifting an object against gravity and resisting its pull when you set it back down.

When you stop and think about it, we are just lifting objects through an arbitrary range of motion.

We are not saving the world or being heroic or going "beast mode," or any other hyperbolic term plastered on a meme floating around social media intended to get you psyched up to hit the gym.

Working out is a privilege. Have you ever looked at it that way?

Being a member of a gym, or having a home gym, is a luxury. We do these arbitrary exercises in hopes of becoming healthier, stronger, better versions of ourselves. To physically challenge ourselves and to achieve goals so we discover what we're capable of doing and to live a higher-quality life.

But let's not delude ourselves into thinking it's anything more than that. Let's keep these activities in perspective. This isn't intended to belittle the act of working out or self-care. Rather, looking at the simple reality of what we're doing should help remove the unnecessary stress, frustration, and confusion that oftentimes gets mixed in with it. See it clearly for what it is, and what it is not, and you'll have freedom to enjoy it.

When you move your body today, whether you lift weights or go for a walk, remind yourself that the activity is a privilege. And how does that renewed perspective make you feel or view the activity?

Day 14
THE NAKED TRUTH, PART II.

Have you ever said something like, "I was bad for eating that dessert"?

The pervasive diet culture has led countless individuals to develop disordered eating habits. In particular, the "clean" and "dirty" food dichotomy has captured many in its grip, causing them to associate their self-worth with food choices.

A helpful exercise to break this unfortunate association between food choices and self-worth is to try to strip food of any emotional attachments that have been formed over the years, and look directly at its individual ingredients.

A homemade chocolate chip cookie is not *bad* or *sinful* or *cheating*, or any other term cloaked in a negative connotation. It is a combination of flour, butter, sugar, salt, baking soda, and chocolate chips. That is all it is. While it is calorically dense and not a good source of nutrition, eating it does not make you a bad person. Shame and guilt from eating cookies are not included in the ingredient list; they're added by us.

A perfectly roasted chicken breast (or vegan-friendly option like tofu, if you prefer) is not *good* or *virtuous*. It is a piece of animal flesh (or block of plant-based matter). That is all. While it is nutritious, it doesn't make you a better person for eating it.

Begin to remove the emotional, subjective element that clings to your food choices. Look at food and see *what it is*, and what it is not. Be aware of the hyperbolic language used to describe it: "This chocolate chip cookie is *sinfully* good and I shouldn't eat it because I'll be 'cheating' on my diet and that would make me 'bad,'" should simply be, "This is a chocolate chip cookie, and I'm going to enjoy it."

Do you often attach judgments about yourself to your food

choices? Do you call yourself "good" for eating certain foods and "bad" for enjoying others? Try to break the bond that may have formed between food and what you think about yourself for eating it. What you eat shouldn't lead to personal judgments.

Day 15

BEWARE OF CONSTANTLY CHASING "MORE."

There's an unfortunate detour many inadvertently end up traveling once they've begun a health and fitness journey. They're motivated by the results they achieve—their clothes fit better, they feel incredible, they enjoy their workouts, maybe they've shed excess weight, they're much stronger.

Then they want, or demand, *more*.

They want to get leaner.

They want to look even better.

They want to improve a specific body part.

They want to lift even more weight for more reps.

They want the number on the scale to keep decreasing.

They want to set bigger personal records.

Every time a goal is reached, they immediately set their sights on the *next* body part or trait to "improve," or personal record to chase, not realizing this path is the shortcut to constant dissatisfaction.

There's nothing wrong with setting new goals or rewarding challenges—they give your training purpose and bring a tremendous sense of accomplishment as you attain them. However, don't overlook *what you've already achieved*. Enjoy what you've already accomplished. Don't be in such a rush to achieve "more" that you neglect to savor the victories you've attained. (Keep in mind *maintaining* results you've achieved is a tremendous victory, too.)

Relentlessly chasing "more" and "better" in the absence of enjoying the journey and being proud of all you've achieved is a sure path to discontentment.

Do you constantly think about the next goal that will "improve" your body and make you happier, or a new personal record you want to set? Take time to record the goals and benefits you've already achieved. Even the seemingly small wins add up to great achievements.

Day 16
NOT A TYPICAL FOOD CHALLENGE, PART I.

We love food. We love food so much we talk about the next delicious meal we want to enjoy *while we're eating an amazing meal*. The irony is that we may not fully enjoy the meal in front of us because we're thinking about what delicious meal we'd like to have next.

Maybe you eat in the car while driving the kids around, or grab something quick on the way to work. Maybe you eat while watching a favorite sitcom or with your phone in your hand.

Do you ever actually pay attention to what you're eating? Do you savor it and notice the different textures and tastes? Or do you scarf it down so quickly you end up eating too much and feel overly full because your body didn't have enough time to realize it would've been satisfied from less food?

Today's food challenge is simple: Slow down when you eat your meals and snacks.

Savor the food. Take time to look at it, smell it, and enjoy it *free from distractions*. Don't watch TV or scroll through social media. Eating the meal should be its own experience. Sadly, this is becoming a foreign experience in our culture, since most of us have our faces glued to an electronic device when we eat. Enjoy the meal with company if you'd like, but don't let a TV or other electronic distraction be involved. Once you've finished eating, sit there a few minutes, or get up and do something else. Pay attention to how you feel. Are you satisfied? Too full? Use that feedback next time you eat.

Day 17
NOT A TYPICAL FOOD CHALLENGE, PART II.

Starting today, and for the next seven days, record everything you eat and drink. You don't need to track the calories or macronutrients (grams of fat, protein, carbohydrates), but be specific about the foods and beverages. For example, don't just record *coffee* if you take your coffee with a spoonful of sugar and cream. Write down *coffee with a spoonful of sugar and cream*. Don't just record *chicken salad* if your chicken salad also includes lots of dressing, cheese, croutons, and bacon.

Pay attention to how you feel after meals and record that information, too; you can even record *why* you ate certain foods. Perhaps you had increased energy, or felt too full after a huge dinner. Maybe you were hungry soon after enjoying a favorite candy bar. Maybe you were bored and rummaged through the cabinets for something crunchy to eat. Write it all down. This information will come in handy eight days from now.

Use an app on your phone, a journal, or whatever you prefer. Just start recording today. Record all foods and beverages, even small bites and sips.

Important! This is a judgment- and guilt-free exercise. Your food choices do not make you "good" or "bad"; this exercise will simply reveal exactly what you eat and drink regularly. This is an objective collection of data, nothing more.

The act of physically recording these things may unveil what you don't see when relying solely on memory.

Day 18

PUNISHMENT OR PRIVILEGE?

Do you go to the gym to punish yourself for packing on weight over the years, or to "work off" that candy bar you ate yesterday? Do you force yourself to eat plain salads and bland chicken breasts as a punishment for going off your diet over the weekend? Do you say things like "I look terrible—I need to work out more often"?

Or do you work out because you're worth the self-care investment? Do you work out because you enjoy the challenge and love seeing how strong you can become? Do you eat minimally-processed foods you enjoy because they're satisfying and make you feel great and are a short- and long-term investment in your health and well-being?

Moving your body. Eating satisfying, nutrient-dense foods. These actions can be a punishment or a privilege. You get to choose. Today, what will be your reasons for eating the foods you choose? Why will you move your body? How will you make nutrition and fitness the privilege it is meant to be?

Day 19
THE POWER OF PERSPECTIVE.

Imagine you were just told you had one week to live. Countless thoughts would flash through your mind. Things you've done; things you *wish* you would've done; people you love; heart-warming memories.

Reaching a certain number on the bathroom scale or building the perfect backside wouldn't even crack the top one hundred thoughts pulsing through your mind. They likely would *never* enter your mind. Yet we can spend ample time each day preoccupied with thoughts about food, our bodies, our workouts.

The main purpose of health and fitness should be—must be—to help you live your best life.

The moment each one of us is born, our life's hourglass hits the table and begins the countdown of our existence. Each grain of sand that falls means another moment closer to our inevitable expiration.

This reality shouldn't cause anxiety or melancholy. It should be sobering. It should bring clarity about what matters to us, and the abundance that doesn't (someone made a rude comment about us, we chose deep-fried tater tots instead of a salad, our butt doesn't look "perfect" in our jeans) but that we allow to preoccupy our minds and distract us.

Is getting six-pack abs *really* what you want? If so, get it done and be sure to enjoy the process required to make that happen. Or do you want your body to serve you and your other goals? Do you want a lifestyle that improves your quality of life and overall health, and allow results like less body fat to be a side effect from that higher purpose?

Today, as you ruminate on who and what matter most to you, think about the role you want health and fitness to play in your life. What do you want it to do for you?

Day 20
THE ESSENTIALS.

Strip away the hype, the noise, the outright nonsense, the inflated sense of self-righteousness and superiority that so often cling to messages of health and fitness ... what would remain?

What *really* matters in the health and fitness pursuit? What are the non-negotiable essentials to improving health and changing one's body?

Moving your body. Consistently, in whatever ways *you enjoy* and prefer, and will adhere to long term.

Nourishing your body with mostly minimally-processed, nutrient-dense foods. Consistently, in whatever method you enjoy and can adhere to long term.

Notice what isn't there. No applause from others; no deprivation or misery; no motivational hashtags; no provocative pictures; no one-size-fits-all approach; no complication; no guilt or obsession; no useless and overpriced supplements.

It's easy to think a fitness journey is time consuming, stressful, and complicated. This is especially true in today's social-media obsessed world where fitness is sensationalized. It's gone from being a tool of self-improvement to a religion where each congregation claims their workout and eating style is supreme and divine.

But when you shatter the façade and stare directly at the bare essentials of what truly defines a health and fitness regimen, what becomes visible is the simplicity. Move your body frequently in ways you enjoy. Eat plenty of whole foods, while including room for your favorite not-super-healthy foods, too. Adherence to these principles is essential for success, so they must be as simple and enjoyable as possible.

Strip away the distracting nonessentials. What you are left with are a few *actions* that should be taken. Actions that should turn into lifelong habits that must be tailored to fit your lifestyle and preferences.

What are some of the distractions you've encountered on your journey? Are there any you need to discard right now? What are two or three essential actions you can take consistently that will develop, or strengthen, your health and fitness journey?

Days 21-30

Day 21

CUT THE STRINGS.

If you're like most women, you may think you operate with high autonomy on a daily basis.

You decide what you will do, how you will do it, why you will do it.

And yet, if you're offered a couple cookies, you don't stop and think, "Am I hungry? Do I really want these? Will I enjoy them, or am I eating them because they're in front of me?" You feel the tug of a string that's long been attached to you—eating food you were offered—and you eat the cookies without any forethought.

Your schedule gets interrupted and you use it as an excuse to skip a workout. This string jerks you—things didn't work out the way you wanted today—and your actions, or lack thereof, go its direction.

You eat pizza and ice cream and feel the familiar tug of guilt, and you begin to bargain with yourself to do an extra workout to "make up for the damage" and vow to diet harder the following day.

These strings are firmly anchored and have the power to jerk you around.

The great news is that once you identify these strings, the ones that have been attached for years or decades and were, perhaps, invisible until now, or identify new ones starting to take hold, then you have the power to cut them and reclaim your autonomy.

As you go about your day, prepare your mind to identify any subtle strings that have their hold on you, and pay attention to the direction they attempt to take you. Then create a plan to cut them.

Day 22
DON'T LISTEN TO YOUR EGO.

Maybe you don't skip a workout even when your routine gets obliterated.

Maybe you're not always tempted by tasty treats that lie around at work or at home.

Maybe one of the thickest strings attached to you that determines your choices and actions, is your ego.

Perhaps your warm-up sets feel heavier than normal, and you notice an ache that increases as the weights get heavier, but you're determined to improve your performance. You *must* do better than the last time you performed the workout. Not improving or, worse, not at least *matching* your previous performance, is a failure.

So you push forward. Even though it was ugly and felt horrible, you forced yourself to do better than last time. Rather than finishing the workout feeling proud and strong, you feel depleted and have a nagging ache that lingers into the following days.

Maybe life stress has had a recent upswing, but you refuse to adjust your workouts despite losing sleep and your workout performance taking a dip. You continue pushing as hard as ever, determined to make progress, refusing to allow circumstances to affect your regimen. But eventually the accumulation of stress builds up and your workout performance stalls, and then regresses.

Just like giving in to the whim of eating every tasty treat that crosses your path isn't in your best interest, neither is giving your ego free rein to dictate your decisions.

Your ego has no place in your workout routine.

Don't let your pride get in the way of smart training. Respect whatever circumstances arise, be as *objective* as you can in handling them. If you experience an ache or discomfort with an exercise, you could limit the weights for the day to the amount that allows you to perform the exercise without discomfort, or you could swap it out for a similar variation if the original exercise didn't feel great. During high-stress times, as another example, you could work out three days per week instead of four, or cut down the total training volume (perform 1-2 fewer sets per exercise) or intensity (leave 3-4 reps "in the tank" at the end of every set).

Your ego can make bad choices and steer you in the wrong direction. Take back the reins.

Do you have a tendency to let your ego take over, or can you recall a time when you gave it control? What were the consequences of that choice and, knowing what you know now, what could you have done instead?

Day 23
THE POWER OF A PAUSE.

"Between stimulus and response there is a space. In that space is our power to choose our response. In our response lies our growth and freedom."
–Viktor Frankl, Holocaust survivor and author of *Man's Search for Meaning*

There's tremendous power in those fleeting moments between a stimulus and your response to it. You just don't realize it's there. You might think A (an event) causes B (your response) to occur, but there's a tiny space between A and B where your choice of response lies.

Grab hold of that space. Use it.

Think about your frequent struggles, or a habit you'd like to change. Do you quickly devour any food lying around at work? Do you often skip workouts? Do you order an extra-large meal at the drive through on the way home after a stressful day? Do you respond immediately with negative comments when you catch your reflection in the mirror or see yourself in photos?

Rehearse the most common events in your mind. Identify the stimulus (e.g., someone brings sweets into the office, or you see yourself in a photo) and your usual response (you mindlessly eat the sweets, or immediately make a negative comment about your body, respectively). Now stop and think about the tiny space that separates the stimulus and your response. The instant right before you act. *That* is when you get to decide the response you will choose.

Next time you encounter that same event, immediately when you face the stimulus, grab hold of that moment before your response, and choose who you want to be in that instant.

Day 24
IF IT'S IMPORTANT, IT WILL TAKE TIME.

"Nothing important comes into being overnight; even grapes or figs take time to ripen. If you say that you want a fig now, I will tell you to be patient."

–Epictetus

Those words from Epictetus are as true now as they were two thousand years ago when presented during one of his lectures. Not much has changed with humanity in the past centuries, or millenniums.

We're an impatient species and whatever we desire—less belly fat, a larger bank account, new car, college degree, the meal you've ordered at a restaurant—we do not like waiting a long time to get it.

Aside from the few that have won the genetic lottery, the people you see in the gym who are the strongest, leanest, or subjectively have "the best physique" didn't get to that point in just a single year, much less in a couple months.

When you catch yourself surrendering to impatience, getting frustrated that you aren't seeing or feeling changes as quickly as you'd like, remind yourself that great things, important things, take time.

You'll make progress if you keep going. You'll enjoy it more too if you can muster up some patience. When you catch yourself getting impatient, remind yourself that great things take time, and once you attain them, they'll taste even sweeter because of the effort they demanded.

Day 25

YOUR HAPPINESS IS NOT CONDITIONAL.

"I'll be happy when I finally lose this weight." "I'll be happy when I can lift the weights I was able to lift a couple years ago." Have you ever said something similar?

You don't have to wait until you improve your health or strength or endurance, or alter your physical appearance, to be happy. If you can't find a way to be happy as you are now, what makes you think you'll be happy then? Be honest—won't you just find something else to "fix" or "improve" when you attain the goal you're currently allowing to hold your happiness captive?

You have every right to lose weight, build muscle, get stronger, or change the appearance of your body so you'll feel more confident, have more energy to go about daily life, or any other reason you want to do it. If your health isn't currently as good as it could be, getting on a path of health improvement is a worthy pursuit.

Do not allow your happiness and confidence to hinge on attainment of that goal, be it losing excess weight, building a toned-looking body, achieving a better blood panel, or reaching a level of performance you previously were capable of.

Find enjoyment in the journey—the *actions* themselves that will produce the desired outcome. Choose to see each workout as its own reward. Take time to discover simple meals you can prepare (or buy) that nourish you and satisfy your taste buds.

Think about your main goal. How can you be happier today, right where you are? What can you do to find enjoyment with your workouts? Your meals?

Day 26
NOT SOMEDAY. TODAY.

Imagine the "after" photo you have in mind that you want to attain from your health and fitness regimen.

We practically foam at the mouth lusting over the "after" photos we envision as we embark on a new workout program. We imagine a flatter stomach; sliding into a smaller (or larger) pant size; less cellulite on our thighs; more muscle on our butts; renewed self-confidence.

Obsessing over the "after" is a mistake that can lead to a by-any-means-necessary attitude. This is what tempts people into trying restrictive fad diets that are not only unsustainable, but are inaccurate with their claims. Any diet that claims to be "best" or "superior" for weight loss is nonsense—research has shown that any diet that creates a negative energy balance leads to weight loss. There is no single best diet for everyone.[1] There is only what is best for *you*. One person may love eating a low-carb diet, someone else may do better with higher carbohydrates and less fat. Another person may prefer a vegetarian diet. Don't feel obligated to try the latest diet craze if you know it'll be unsustainable or unenjoyable (i.e., don't follow a low-carb diet if you like carb-rich foods).

Too many people want to blast through the time between their "before" and the elusive "after" just to get the process over with. If you try to just get it over with to reach the "after" state, you either won't achieve it, or won't maintain it for long.

What about *after* the "after"? If you don't find a way to enjoy the process it takes to get there—to build habits you can adhere to—you won't be able to maintain the results you achieve. Your

---

[1]. Rachel Freire Ph.D., "Scientific Evidence of Diets for Weight Loss: Different Macronutrient Composition, Intermittent Fasting, and Popular Diets," Nutrition (January 2020), https://www.sciencedirect.com/science/article/pii/S0899900719301030.

health and fitness journey shouldn't be about achieving an "after" version of yourself as quickly as possible, but creating an enjoyable journey that leads to the results you want, while ensuring you *maintain* them well into the future.

Ultimately, this journey shouldn't have a finish line. It should be a lifelong pursuit.

"Can I keep doing this thing for months and years?" is a question worth asking before making a change to your eating and workout habits. If the answer is "No," look for an action or change you can enthusiastically say "Yes!" to.

Day 27
A BETTER BEFORE AND AFTER.

Yesterday, the "before and after" people seek from a new workout regimen was discussed. Have you noticed that the only before and after images shown, and sought, are exclusively about physical appearance? Drastic weight loss; clothing sizes dropped; inches shed; curves added to the "right" places on the body.

As usual in the health and fitness world, how you look is touted as the most important factor. Your success is based solely on the physical "after" transformation you do or do not achieve.

You deserve more than that. You should *demand* more than that.

What results could be equally as important (arguably more so) than being leaner/lighter/more attractive/curvier?

- Feeling good about yourself
- Fewer aches and pains
- Performing tasks of daily living with greater ease
- Increased bone density
- Improvements in blood pressure and other health markers
- Not obsessing over food
- Greater self-confidence
- Developing, or further solidifying, a workout habit
- Physical strength and stamina
- Shattering self-imposed limitations

You could continue adding to that list, no doubt, and you should.

As you continue your health and fitness journey, thinking about the "after" is okay, but set your sights on something more meaningful than just looking good. In fact, by striving to attain the benefits listed above, you'll find yourself looking better as a side effect.

Day 28
NOT A TYPICAL FOOD CHALLENGE, PART III.

Seven days ago, you started a food journal and recorded everything you ate and drank for a week. Perhaps you even analyzed why you ate and how you felt afterward.

Most who perform this exercise for the first time quickly discover they don't eat quite like they thought. Maybe a few more sweets or sodas snuck in there than you realized. Maybe you noticed that on days you skipped breakfast, you were more likely to overeat later in the day. Maybe you have the habit of snacking when you're bored. Maybe you don't eat as many fruits and vegetables as you thought you did. Maybe you consume a lot of calorie-dense beverages.

Remember, this exercise was not meant to elicit an emotional response, either good or bad, or lead to judgment about yourself. The goal was simply to make you aware of your habits and the totality of your average food choices.

Did you discover where simple improvements can be made? Perhaps you could eat more minimally-processed foods (e.g.: oatmeal or whole wheat bread instead of crackers), increase protein intake (e.g.: low-fat dairy, lean meats, fish, tofu/edamame), eat more fiber-rich foods, eat breakfast so you're not ravenous and end up overeating later. You could add more vegetables and fruits to your meals, swap out sugary beverages for calorie-free options, or choose to go for a walk or read a book when the urge to mindlessly snack beckons. Now that you know how you typically eat during a week, you know exactly what can be done.

Small modifications add up over time. If you see there is room for some improvement with your nutrition habits, start there.

Remember, making room for your favorite foods is important, too. This is a lifestyle you're building, and your favorite foods should be part of it. Don't just think about what should be *limited*—focus on what can be *added*.

What surprised you or where would you like to make simple and sustainable changes? How will you use this knowledge going forward?

Day 29

WHAT DO YOU NEED TO DO NEXT?

It happens to the best of us. We *know* feeling guilty doesn't ameliorate a recent event, nor help us move past it.

Still, whatever frequent battle you fight—overeating, skipping workouts, negative self-talk, being controlled by the number on the bathroom scale, comparing your body to the woman at the gym, giving your ego the reins, obsessing over changing the appearance of your body, making not-so-healthy food choices for days at a time, feeling guilty when you enjoy a favorite food—it may conclude with you being engulfed in a shame storm.

Feeling confused, frustrated, or overwhelmed with guilt, wanting to do the "right" thing but struggling to take that step (or figure out what that first step should be), is not a fun mental game to play, because you can't win.

When you find yourself in this territory you need only to ask yourself one question: What do I need to do next?

It doesn't need to be anything complicated or extravagant. In fact, make it as simple as possible, *then do it immediately.* Stop trying to think your way out of the problem. Instead, come up with a simple action to take, so you can move past it.

You can change the momentum with the next meal, next workout, next thought, next journal entry.

What do you need to do next?

Day 30
WHEN IT ALL GOES UP IN FLAMES.

One evening after dinner, inventor Thomas Edison was told his business facility was on fire. He arrived at the scene to witness fire engines, hundreds of spectators, and flames soaring seven stories high, engulfing *years* of his groundbreaking research, prototypes, and records.

An enormous amount of time and effort and discovery, a life's culmination of work, incinerated in an instant. Lost forever.

Amidst the fiery chaos, Edison found his son and told him to get his mother and her friends: "They'll never see a fire like this again!" His son looked at him dumbfounded, understandably, to which Edison responded, "It's all right. We've just got rid of a lot of rubbish."

Edison admired an inferno that consumed his life's work, groundbreaking research, and millions of dollars of investments. You get upset (as we all do) when someone cuts you off in traffic; when the store is out of your favorite produce; when someone hogs a piece of equipment at the gym; when a coworker takes the last cup of coffee and doesn't make a fresh pot; when you don't improve your performance from last week.

Some events in our lives can be labeled as catastrophic. Many more are not, thankfully, yet we treat them as if they were.

What if you could reframe events—even those that result in loss or extreme inconvenience—as opportunities instead of disasters? Can you choose to be "rid of a lot of rubbish" instead of choosing to feel annoyed or inconvenienced?

Days 31–40

Day 31
LIKE AN INVESTMENT.

Every workout you do, each nourishing meal you eat, each not-super-healthy meal or food you eat *guilt free*, each moment of awareness on your thoughts and mindset—these are investments in your health and self-care. Over time they compound, providing dividends.

Just as depositing money into a savings account or investing in a Roth IRA leads to growth that compounds over time, so too do your repeated actions involving food, fitness, and mindfulness.

The workouts you did this week? You just issued a few deposits into your long-term health account.

That lunch you packed that kept you satisfied all afternoon while delivering a couple servings of veggies and protein? That's another deposit.

Catching yourself staring at a part of your body you don't love, but refusing to escalate the old *I-don't-like-that* conversation, and instead choosing to focus on what your body allows you *to do* that you're grateful for? Another deposit that will continue paying dividends now, and into the future.

Some of these investments provide immediate benefits—that workout will make you feel great today and that meal will aid in recovery and provide nourishment. Some will need to be powered by repetition—weeks and months of consistent training will increase your strength, build muscle, boost fat loss. And some have greater effects over the long term—quality of life, stave off disease, build bone density.

What deposits will you make today? This week?

Day 32
AVOID DISTRACTIONS.

Have you ever tried a new diet or workout program because someone swore by its results? Or you overhead someone discussing their new diet and wondered, "Could this be the solution I've been waiting for?"

Another is raving about their new workout program and you inquire, hoping this will finally help you achieve the bodily changes you crave. A friend or social media icon says a new powdered drink mix helped her lose weight and reduce cravings and improve energy levels and help her sleep better. (Big news! You can too! Discount code in bio.)

You *know* what sounds too good to be true usually is, but you can't help having your curiosity tugged by the possibility of fast results. It is, after all, human nature to desire an easier path, faster and more noticeable results with less effort required on your part. These *You can lose 10 pounds fast and never crave sugar again!* promises are akin to get-rich-quick schemes that lure you in with hyperbolic promises of making a quick buck with zero effort or risk.

These tempting claims are distractions, and nothing more. It's the same recycled nonsense; that's why fads and many supplements come and go, because none of them are as incredible as they claim to be. Eventually they fizzle out, and something else takes their place.

The solution? Ignore distractions like pills, powders, supplements, gimmicks, fads, secrets, hacks, weight-loss wraps. Stick to the proven basics and master them.

Are you:

- Eating mostly whole foods and getting sufficient protein (0.7 to 1 gram per pound of bodyweight) and fiber (approximately 25-30 grams per day)?
- Getting adequate sleep most nights?
- Exercising regularly?
- Managing stress?
- Avoiding smoking and drugs?

Do you:

- Practice moderation with alcohol?
- Successfully catch yourself calling certain foods "good" and "bad" and aim to remove those unhelpful dichotomous labels because you know food is just food?
- Have meaningful and rewarding relationships?

Those things are proven to improve health, so that is where your efforts should be focused, not on the expensive, unproven, embellished promises of fad supplements and products that prey on insecurities and desires for immediate results.

Which of those basics have you mastered? Which could you improve? Nothing will overshadow them, and no supplement can replace them.

Day 33
BEWARE OF THE (FALSE) GUILT-FREE TRAP.

Myriad recipes beginning with "guilt free" in the title are popular.

Guilt-free brownies. Guilt-free pizza and pasta. All recipes intended to be healthier versions of the original they seek to revamp, and because they're (supposedly) healthier they've been labeled as "guilt free" to boot.

"You don't need to feel guilty for eating these brownies because they're made with beans and honey and coconut oil!" they proclaim.

This *but-it's-healthy* halo can lead to the justification that it's okay to eat multiple servings of the food at once. After all, it's *healthy*. This can create its own problems like promoting overeating and further strengthening the good/bad food dichotomy that can lead to a bad relationship with how you view food.

Here's a radical idea: Every single food, every single recipe, regardless of its ingredients, should be enjoyed guilt free.

Sugar-laden and high-fat brownies? You can eat one and not feel guilty.

"Healthier" brownies made with beans and avocado? You can eat one and not feel guilty. Or innocent.

Remember, guilt and innocence are never in the ingredients list. Do yourself a favor and remove all claims of morality from your food choices and abolish the good/bad dichotomy that many sources have attached to food. Do away with self-professed guilty-pleasure foods while you're at it.

When did you last find yourself in the guilt-free recipe trap, and can you see how that mindset isn't helpful?

Day 34
PURPOSE. NOT PASSION.

Most people rely on passion as the fuel source to power them toward their goals. They want to "feel like" doing the necessary things. They want to *feel like* going to the gym first thing in the morning. They want to *feel like* choosing nourishing meals instead of the tempting not-so-healthy options. They want to *feel like* saying no to dessert.

Passion oftentimes is the catalyst that initially spurs us into action. When faced with real-life obstacles, however—time constraints, hobbies, your kid's activities, work projects—passion vanishes; it's no match for the daily conditions we must maneuver. No longer fueled by the passion-driven *feel likes*, we stop.

The problem, you see, is that passion is a temporary, feel-good emotion. It's fleeting and finite. As such, it's an inadequate fuel source for achieving your goals.

Purpose, however, is a must-complete mission. It is what sustains you in the absence of motivation. Purpose propels you forward even when you don't *feel like* taking action. Investing in your health is a purpose; getting stronger is a purpose; doing something just for you is a purpose; strengthening a healthy habit is a purpose; building a routine that makes you the best version of yourself is a purpose.

When you're tempted to skip a workout or prepare your meals for the week because you don't *feel like* doing it, don't anxiously wait for passion to return. Shift your focus to a worthy purpose.

What will be the purpose that sustains you when you don't "feel like" investing in self-care? What will keep you moving forward instead of halting you in your tracks?

Day 35

ONLY WHAT YOU THINK SHOULD MATTER.

Dolly Parton is an iconic figure. Regardless of your opinion about her music or personal style, one thing is certain: She doesn't care what you or anyone else thinks about her.

Her trademark persona was inspired, in her own words, by the town tramp. Parton wasn't exposed to movie stars in magazines and movies in her small Tennessee hometown. To her, the local prostitute was beautiful and looked like a movie star.

Everyone thought she was joking, saying the prostitute was trash. Parton's response was, "That is what I am going to grow up to be—trash." She chose to emulate the styling of a prostitute and didn't care if people thought she was joking or utterly ridiculous. The only opinion that mattered to Dolly Parton was her own.

How much merit do you give to other people's opinions? If you're like most people, it's too much. You care more about their opinions about how you look, what you wear, how you live your life than about what really makes you happy.

What's the problem with this? It means you relinquish your control, allowing the opinions of others to dictate your choices. You do the things they want you to do, because you crave their approval. You don't do the things you want to do, in fear of their disapproval.

Where does that get you? Looking to the opinions of others to shape your actions is akin to being batted around like a tennis ball. You go whatever direction the rackets dictate; you're simply along for the ride.

It's not always easy to know who you are and who you want to be. But if your general goal is to be a good person with sound values flavored with characteristics and personality that make you unique, why should anyone else's opinion matter?

Regardless of what you do, whether it's being true to yourself or submitting to the assumed roles you think others want you to adopt, there will always be people who don't approve. You can never please everyone.

Why not focus on being the person you approve of?

Day 36

DO NOT FEAR FAILURE.

You took a chance, tried a new approach, finally pushed yourself out of your comfort zone, did what you thought was truly best … and failed.

When failure happens, especially when it's preceded by a tremendous amount of time and effort, we may quickly label ourselves a failure. We take on the *I am a failure* proclamation as part of our identity, like a thread woven into the fabric of our being.

That's the wrong response. The failure was an *experience*. It does not define you as a person.

You decide what the failure will mean.

Will you perceive the experience as an invaluable learning opportunity, refusing to squander the real-life education it provides? Will you choose to assess the event and confront, as objectively as possible, what happened and why? Will you consider, "What could I have done differently" or, perhaps, "How will I use this information going forward to better prepare myself"?

Or will you feel sorry for yourself, allow the experience to prevent you from trying again, and give the event the power to cripple you and stunt your growth?

You have two options when it comes to failure:

1. Embrace it as an *experience* and commit to learning from it.

2. Embrace it as an identity and give it power to prevent you from learning, growing, and achieving your goals.

Life is full of failures. (If it's not, that means you're not actively trying.) Some are small like a firecracker, quick to fizzle out. Others may explode with such tremendous force that you're instantly knocked on your butt, left stunned and dazed.

We all fail, and we can choose our responses to those events, and determine how they will make us better, or worse.

Think about a recent failure. Did you initially see it as an experience or something that defined you? How can you view it as a learning opportunity, and how can you use that perspective going forward?

Day 37

SUPPORTING OR UNDERMINING?

Is this supporting and helping create the lifestyle I want, or is it undermining my goals?

Use that question as a lens through which to view your habits and actions.

Do you want a health and fitness lifestyle that empowers you, makes you feel great about yourself, helps you achieve your goals, is free from obsession and guilt, and enhances your life rather than dominating it? Then pay attention to what you do and think, and see if those thoughts and actions support or undermine those goals.

Doing an abbreviated workout because your workout window got slashed from one hour to 30 minutes? Supporting.

Defining foods dichotomously (good/bad) and choosing to feel guilty for eating your favorite dessert because you've labeled it a "bad" food? Undermining.

Allowing fear to prevent you from going to "that part" of the gym, learning new exercises, pushing yourself to see what you're capable of doing? Undermining.

Going completely off your plan for a week by missing workouts and not eating mostly nutrient-dense foods, but choosing to respond with self-compassion, examining *why* that happened and creating a simple-to-execute plan going forward? Supporting.

Demanding perfection from yourself instead of executing the most important actions consistently, realizing what you do most often over the long term is what matters most? Undermining.

Using extreme restriction or extra workouts to punish yourself for not seeing changes on the scale? Undermining.

Creating new health and fitness goals that allow you to appreciate your body for what it's capable of doing and achieving? Supporting.

If the goal is a health and fitness *lifestyle* free from obsession, deprivation, unnecessary stress and is defined by empowerment, enjoyment, life enhancement, flexibility, then be mindful of your thoughts and actions, and ensure they are supporting that goal. If they're not, replace them with something that will support you. As for the thoughts and actions you're currently doing that support your goals, continue repeating and replicating them.

Day 38
FAT LOSS IS NOT THE ONLY OPTION.

Despite the eye-grabbing headlines on mainstream magazines and the FitSpo messages commanding social media, you can seek to improve your nutrition and workout habits for reasons other than fat loss or "fixing" parts of your body.

If your experiences with changing your eating and workout habits were done exclusively for the purpose of shedding excess fat or improving the appearance of your body, then you may be elated at what you discover when you shift your focus to something else.

Try a different approach. Have reasons other than losing weight or fixing "flaws" to tweak your nutrition choices and exercise habits.

- Improve health markers (e.g.: blood pressure, cholesterol)
- Get stronger by lifting heavier barbells and dumbbells
- Increase your endurance and work capacity
- Manage stress
- Alleviate aches and pains

There are dozens of other reasons you can choose to perform a workout or establish health-promoting eating habits.

If you're mentally exhausted from a years- or decades-long focus (or obsession) on losing weight or "fixing" your body, take a refreshing and empowering approach for a while. Ask yourself before eating a meal or doing a workout, "What is a great reason to do this that has nothing to do with weight loss or altering the appearance of my body?"

Start collecting your non-scale victories. Today, how many can you tally?

Day 39
NOURISH A GROWTH MINDSET.

There's an unavoidable obstacle in your path. How do you respond? Do you shrink back from the challenge, seeing it as proof that you "don't have it in you" to make progress?

Or do you stare down the obstacle, commit to learning a new tactic or skill until you overcome it?

The former response would be what Carol Dweck, author of *Mindset: The New Psychology of Success*, calls a fixed mindset (seeing criticism or challenges as proof you don't have the necessary abilities). The latter response, on the other hand, is a growth mindset (the necessary skills or abilities to face and overcome challenges can be cultivated and built).

Someone with a fixed mindset may try to improve their nutrition, but quickly find themselves back to old habits. "I just can't stick to diet changes!" they say. It would benefit this individual to realize change *is* possible. They shouldn't continue repeating the same ineffective strategies, if that's why they were unsuccessful, but should instead try different approaches until they find one that works better for them.

By contrast, someone with a growth mindset may try a new style of eating, but also find themselves quickly reverting to old habits. Rather than saying they can never stick to diet changes, they assess what happened and instead of trying the same ineffective routine again, they look to a new approach that's better suited to their lifestyle, personality, and preferences. In other words, something they can more easily adhere to. They know change is possible; they just may need to try a few things first to find what's best for them.

Know that skills can be cultivated, and obstacles can be opportunities. Failure is not definitive and shouldn't stop you from trying again. Raw talent isn't necessary; instead, consistent analysis and effort are keys to success.

Nourish a growth mindset by reminding yourself of those truths. Where do you most need to apply that knowledge, and how will you do so today?

Day 40
WHY ARE WE NEVER SATISFIED? PART I.

"I'll be happy when I have …" we tell ourselves.

Think about something you wanted for years, something you had to work hard to achieve. You saved money, bit by bit, until you had enough to buy that car, that house, that new piece of home gym equipment, take a vacation, go back to school, found a relationship.

And yet, not too long after you finally got what you wanted, did you *want more*? Perhaps something even better?

In *A Guide to the Good Life*, psychologists Shane Frederick and George Loewenstein coined the term "hedonic adaptation." It states that we want something, we work hard to fulfill the desire, but once we finally have it or satisfied the craving, we desire something else. And the whole process starts again.

Once we attain our desire, we adapt to its presence and stop desiring it, or simply don't enjoy it as much as we did initially. We're again bored or just as dissatisfied as we were before getting it, and seek the next thing or experience to satisfy our renewed craving.

The same cycle—have a desire, work hard to fulfill it, experience momentary joy, the initial excitement and appreciation wanes, seek something newer and better—happens with health and fitness too. (More on that tomorrow.)

Reflect on something, whether it was an experience, a milestone event in your life or career, or an item you purchased, that you worked hard and patiently to earn. How long were you satisfied with it? When did you grow used to its presence and experience a decrease in satisfaction, and what did you desire next?

This exercise can be powerful when we find a pattern that repeats itself, because then we can figure out *why* we do it. Knowing why empowers us to change it, or at least drain some of its power.

Days 41-50

Day 41
WHY ARE WE NEVER SATISFIED? PART II.

"I'll be happy when I lose this excess weight," the woman who lived with obesity for years may say. Through persistent effort, she reached a bodyweight that improved her health and self-confidence, and eradicated aches and pains she dealt with for years.

She may exclaim, "Yes! I did it!" and celebrate her achievement for a time. Soon after, though, she starts lamenting the loose skin on her body. She compares her physique to others at the gym and decides she wants more muscle definition. Gone is the pride she felt from achieving her initial weight loss goal. She's no longer satisfied. "I'll *finally* be happy when this loose skin is gone, and my butt is firmer and perkier."

Don't rely on specific outcomes to determine your satisfaction with your health and body. Don't overlook what you've already achieved. Don't get stuck on the endless rollercoaster of chasing something "better." That's a one-way trip to chronic dissatisfaction.

Go after your goals, especially if they're motivating. Eat more nutritious foods and less "junk" foods; establish habits that define the life you want to live; get stronger; lose weight to improve your health; build a body you feel great occupying; improve your work capacity and endurance; discover what your body is capable of doing; banish the fear of specific foods that only makes them more irresistible.

Having goals is good, and you can and should do whatever you want with your body. Just beware of the trap that leaves you constantly craving *more* out of chronic dissatisfaction and the nagging compulsion that you must always be "improving" or "enhancing" or "fixing" some part of your body or life.

As you achieve your health, fitness, performance, and physique goals, be mindful of the *more-will-make-me-happy* trap. Don't be one of the individuals who says, "I've reached a healthy bodyweight!" only to shrug off the results she worked so hard to achieve and say, "But I don't look good enough yet. Maybe I'll finally be happy when I …"

What achievements are you overlooking because you're chasing "more" or "better"?

Day 42
WHAT WE TAKE FOR GRANTED.

In our quest to achieve *better* results, reach that "next level" of fitness or appearance, to *improve* this feature or *fix* that flaw, to conquer that elusive milestone, we quickly forget about all the work we've already put in. The hours at the gym. The dedication to molding new habits. The progress we earned. The strength we forged.

We adapt to their presence, as discussed in the two prior days' readings, and seek out more, better, advanced, next-level lustrous goals.

Not only does this constant chase of "better" create chronic dissatisfaction, but you also end up taking for granted what you've already achieved, what you have in this moment. Things you wouldn't miss unless they were suddenly taken away.

What health, fitness, mindfulness, performance goals have you achieved that you once desired and worked hard to earn? What things have been a pleasant, welcome surprise that you didn't anticipate experiencing?

Don't overlook the work you've done, the milestones you've achieved, or the things you can do right now. It's good to stop occasionally, look back, and say, "Yes, I did *all* of that. I'm grateful for what I have, and what I am capable of doing today."

So, what have you done? What are you grateful for?

Day 43

SELF-FULFILLING PROPHECIES.

How sad it is to think that once you reach the next chronological decade that your life and abilities are severely limited. Unfortunately, you've probably heard so many people say, "I'm too old to do _____" throughout your life that you accept that statement as a fact for yourself, as well.

Maybe you utter other self-fulfilling prophecies such as:

- "I can never stick to a diet."
- "I could never deadlift twice my bodyweight."
- "I have no willpower, motivation, discipline."
- "Now that I have a family and career, I can't do that."

Self-talk statements that begin with "I'm too _____ to do _____" or "I could never do/be/achieve _____" create and solidify self-determined limitations that turn into self-fulfilling prophecies.

This is not to suggest you need to start chanting vapid platitudes; that's equally useless. But you can identify the self-imposed limitations you've set, or have simply come to believe will be your fate because you've heard them your entire life from others. You can refuse to feed those beliefs. You can make them wilt and wither away.

You can actively denounce them, too. The woman who has always said she could never be strong (or the familiar "I'm too old" excuse) can follow a sound strength training program and make tremendous progress. The woman who says she can never lose weight and improve her health can focus on building just one new habit each month. The woman who thinks health and fitness is too confusing and time-consuming can commit to working out three times per week with a focus on improving her performance and start meal-prepping so she has nourishing lunches to take to work.

The great Roman emperor Marcus Aurelius said, "The soul becomes dyed with the color of its thoughts." Remember that when you find yourself saying something that has the power to become a self-fulfilling prophecy.

What self-fulfilling prophecies do you frequently utter? Are they helpful, or hurtful?

Day 44
STUPID ADVICE.

Want to hear some stupid advice? Here it is: *Just love your body.* If hearing those four words actually led to instantaneous results, then no one would struggle with body image issues.

For someone who feels trapped in her body, has struggled to lose weight and keep it off for years, has a negative self-image of her body's shape or size or appearance, or is constantly trying to fix "flaws," being told to *just love her body* isn't the least bit helpful.

Change does not happen that easily. You don't have to drastically go from not loving your body to loving everything about it and not wanting to change a thing. However, you can appreciate it in new ways and, perhaps, that will help you love it more over time, if even in unexpected ways.

Take, for example, the woman who has disliked her thighs for as long as she can remember. She might work on appreciating her thighs for what they can *do*: run, ride a bike, squat progressively heavier weights. By shifting her focus from her thighs' appearance to performance, she has found a positive way to create appreciation for a body part she has struggled to like.

The woman who has stretch marks or loose skin may have to first work on having a neutral perspective of those features. She doesn't have to "love" them, but she can work on progressing from disliking them to seeing them as just part of her body. They can't magically vanish or diminish, and actively disliking those features doesn't change them; it only creates a mental burden for her to bear.

Instead, she can work on *not* having an opinion about those features. If she catches herself glaring at the stretch marks in the mirror and a negative comment is about to roll off her tongue, she can choose instead to say nothing instead of something hurtful.

You shouldn't be expected to "perfect" your body, or even want to. You shouldn't hate your body, either. It's okay to be completely indifferent to parts of yourself. Appreciate as best you can what your body *can do,* and understand it's okay to be indifferent to other features if you can't find something to appreciate about them. But pay attention as you keep progressing—those "indifferent" parts of your body might surprise you with how awesome they can be.

Do you have parts of your body you actively dislike? Instead of disliking a certain part or feature, can you work on being indifferent to it? Or, even better, can you appreciate it for what it can do?

Day 45

YOU DO WHAT YOU DO. WHY?

We all have habits. Perhaps every weekday morning, you wake up to an alarm, stumble to the kitchen for a cup of much-needed coffee, then shower, eat breakfast, take care of the kids, and drive to work.

We do these things without thinking, almost without effort.

Sometimes these habits are extremely useful and health promoting. Perhaps you work out at five in the morning several days per week before everyone else in the house is awake, rain or shine. Maybe you always eat a protein-rich, high-fiber breakfast that sustains you throughout the first part of the day. These habits help you reach, and maintain, your goals. They form the lifestyle that's important to you.

Then there are habits that don't exactly help. Snacking on high-calorie, low-nutrient foods while watching TV late at night. Skipping your evening workout because you "don't feel like it." Turning to food for comfort every time you experience anxiety. Berating yourself when you deviate from your plan.

The good news is habits can be changed. You can turn current habits that aren't helpful into habits that are. You will need to be diligent and patient, but you can do it. As you go about your day, pay close attention to what you do out of rote habit, both the useful and not so useful. Know why you do what you do.

When you notice a habit that doesn't help you get closer to your goals, figure out why you're doing that thing. Then adjust it. Do something else instead.

Do you frequently skip your evening workout? Try doing it first thing in the morning.

Tend to consume too many calories at night while watching

TV? Swap out your usual snack for a low-calorie option, or eat a more satiating meal for dinner.

Eat when you're bored or anxious? Go for a walk, read a book, write down your thoughts in a journal. Do something else instead of grabbing a snack.

Tend to obsess over every tiny detail of your health and fitness regimen? Suffer from "paralysis by analysis" and never actually implement any changes? Identify two to three *big* actions you can take each day, and do them with intense focus and determination.

Some habits can be more difficult than others to change, but it is possible. Create a plan and execute it, making things as easy as you can to implement. Be patient. Persevere. The habits, both good and bad, you have now didn't develop instantly, and neither will the new ones you want to establish.

Day 46
WHAT IS A CONSTANT STRUGGLE?

Maybe you regularly overeat beyond the point of satiety. Maybe you feel like you lose control with a certain food. Maybe you tend to stop working out with the slightest interruption to your schedule. Maybe it feels like the moment you finally build momentum with your fitness regimen, you're frantically putting out one fire after another in your life, so you abandon the routine.

When you start (or restart) your fitness journey, what is a battle you find yourself facing again and again with you usually coming out on what feels like the losing side?

We all have our counterproductive tendencies. When faced with a certain scenario, you respond out of rote habit, taking action seemingly without even thinking. It's a reflex, rather than a rational choice. And when this response is one that does *not* take you the direction you want to go, you label it a bad habit.

Look back at your journey. What is a battle you often face where you make a choice that doesn't help you?

Is it with food? Do you overindulge then quit even trying to improve nutrition choices out of frustration?

Is it with going to the gym? Do you quit with the first indication of adversity, or do you perform workouts/exercises you don't enjoy?

Is it with your mindset? Do you spend more time engaging in self-talk that breaks you down rather than builds you up? Do you set ridiculously high standards that can't be achieved?

Identify a common scenario you struggle with and examine your usual response. *Now create a plan to deal with it more productively next time it occurs.* How can you respond in a manner that keeps you moving forward? Set yourself up to come out the victor next time.

As an example, you overeat certain foods; it feels like you lose control and end up eating too much. Then you make a string of less-than-ideal choices. Plan of action next time you're around this food: Don't eat directly from containers or actively manage portion sizes (commit to not getting seconds, for example). When you get home from the grocery store, put foods you typically overeat into individual serving-size containers. This way, when you want the food, you eat the allotted portion and won't give in to eating more.

Identify a common struggle, then create a plan to better manage it.

Day 47

EMBRACE YOUR NATURAL ABILITIES.

In yesterday's reading, we discussed how everyone has challenges—things that, for some reason, just take you considerable effort and copious amounts of patience to overcome.

But in addition to habitual challenges, you also have natural abilities; strengths, waiting to be magnified.

It's human nature to focus on your faults and shortcomings—things you'd like to improve or change. Because of this, you're quick to dismiss your strengths.

So let's balance it out and focus on your strengths. What do you naturally excel at doing? What are some of your strengths?

Do you regularly go to the gym? Do you prepare nourishing meals for workday lunches? Maybe your strength is unrelated (directly, at least) to health and fitness: Do you excel at time management? Scheduling? Organization? Analyzing data? Are you willing to work harder than most? Are you great at improvising?

If you have trouble pinpointing your strengths, ask someone close to you: a friend, coworker, spouse. Ask them, "What do you think I'm naturally good at doing? What is one of my major strengths?"

Once you identify your strengths, examine them. What is it you do so well? What situations frequently occur where you put this strength to work? Examine the situations that bring out these strengths.

Now ... *find out how to replicate those strengths.* How can you put them to work to help you reach your health and fitness goals? How can you duplicate and expose them more frequently?

Day 48
DON'T DISDAIN GROWING OLDER.

We've all heard women speak with disdain about their birthday; many even lie about their age. There's even the anticipated mid-life crisis—perhaps you've seen people not handle it well, or maybe even had one yourself.

Do not lament getting older. It's futile to complain about grey hair, wrinkles, eyesight that's not as sharp as it once was, aches and pains that linger longer than they did in your youth, and everything else that comes from spending more time on this planet.

Why be miserable about something you cannot prevent or change?

Gripe, groan, and buy all the useless anti-aging supplements and gimmicks you want, but it will not halt time. It certainly won't reverse it. You are going to get older. Your body is going to change.

Why *choose* to be miserable when you can choose to celebrate spending another year on this spinning rock? It is a choice. Hating getting older, despite what some people say, is not "part of being a woman."

Don't be a participant in the birthday-hating ritual so many choose to be part of every year. You know every year it will come. There's nothing you can do to stop it. Complaining about it creates needless anxiety or sadness.

Instead, embrace getting older. When you stop and think about it, what other choice do you really have? You can't fight it, being upset about it achieves nothing, and the only alternative is … well, you know.

Do what you can to age gracefully and ensure you have a high quality of life, because *that* is what you can control. But the rest that comes with it? Don't fight it, and certainly don't exaggerate or obsess about it. It's as useless as spitting on a raging bonfire in attempt to extinguish it.

Day 49
DELIBERATELY INTRODUCE CHAOS INTO YOUR ROUTINE.

You've heard stories of athletes who have pre-game rituals; the same one they've done for years. They eat the same meal before every game, put on their gear and uniform in the same order, perform the same warm-up routine. You can't help but wonder, "What would happen if they *couldn't* do this routine? How would they respond?"

But guess what? You most likely do the same thing. You wake up the same time every day during the week, and leave the house at the same time to take the same route to work. Perhaps you eat the same breakfast every Monday, Tuesday, etc., or go to the gym the same days of the week at the same time.

But what happens when your routine gets obliterated by Real Life Events? Can you pivot and handle it, or does it paralyze you?

Perhaps you can recall a time you started a new fitness routine, one where you were going to the gym, eating well, and making progress. Then you got derailed by Real Life. Because your routine got interrupted, you chose to quit instead of adapt.

Want to do yourself a tremendous favor? Voluntarily introduce chaos into your usual routine. Choose to go to the gym at a different time of day, or simply use different equipment or perform different exercises. Prepare a different meal than you're used to eating in the morning, or get creative with whatever is in the kitchen for dinner. Instead of allocating a full hour to your workout, cut it to 30 minutes.

Why do this? So that when your routine gets unexpectedly obliterated by Real Life, you'll already know how to respond in a productive, pragmatic way. Because you'll have done it before.

The ability to adapt to a less-than-ideal situation is a critical skill to develop, because hurdles and obstacles and daunting challenges come with the gift of life. Might as well train for these events before they happen, so you're prepared to face them when they do.

Today, how can you introduce a little chaos into your usual routine? What is something that would normally throw you completely off your game? Make it happen, and handle it calmly and confidently.

Day 50
ZOOM OUT.

You missed three scheduled workouts due to an illness. *Will I lose the results I've gained? How should I start back with working out? This is exactly what happens once I build momentum—I have the worst luck!*

Or you overate at a social event, enjoying more rich entrees and indulgent desserts than you planned, and follow this up with another day of less-than-ideal food choices. *Why did I overdo it? How much "damage" will this cause?*

In the moment, you might tend to overreact to the situation. You panic about the effects of the circumstances or your lackluster self-control and how those choices will undermine the goals you've set.

When you find yourself in a similar situation, zoom out. Escape the narrow aperture of that day, or even that week, and zoom out. The event, when viewed in a larger span of time like a month or a year, is far less significant. Like pouring a bucket of water into an Olympic swimming pool, it makes no discernible difference.

When an unplanned situation disrupts your workout regimen; when you enjoy a few too many delectable baked goods, don't respond with panic or, worse, guilt. Zoom out. Then get back to your plan. (Or create one you can implement immediately.)

Always remember, the actions you do *most of the time* for a *long period of time* are the ones that matter most. Set your sights on reinforcing the daily habits that ultimately define a healthy lifestyle. Don't get distracted by the occasional events that interrupt your routine. Deal with them as best you can when they happen, or simply *accept them* if that's the only option, then move forward once again.

Do what you can in the moment, maintain a zoomed-out view

to remind yourself it's the accumulation of repeated actions that lead to results and define a lifestyle.

Have you had an experience recently that would benefit from a zoomed-out perspective?

Days 51-60

Day 51
WHAT ARE YOU FEEDING YOURSELF?

Not in the literal eating and drinking sense. Rather, what are you feeding your *mind*? Take inventory of the health and fitness sources and individuals you follow on social media, the websites you regularly visit, the newsletters you're subscribed to. The information you consume will affect you.

Do these individuals and sources build you up, or tear you down? Do they nourish you and make you feel great about yourself or do they attempt to cram you into a one-size-fits-all mold? Do they help or inspire you to reach *your* goals, or is it a nonstop highlight reel that's all about them and their body and their life? Do they use fear-mongering tactics to sell products and push information on you? Do they promote extreme and unsustainable diet or exercise regimens?

Go on a social media/inbox cleanse. Unfollow and unsubscribe from sources that don't help you, especially those that make you feel less than and cause you to feel anxious, critical or unsure about yourself, and sources that declare "*this* is what being fit looks like" that makes you think you must look a certain way/attain a certain shape or bodyweight before you can love yourself.

If you don't actively define what you want your health and fitness lifestyle to be, then the sources you view will do it for you. What you view and read matters; choose wisely.

Today, examine the sources you follow and regularly read. How does that information make you feel? Rid yourself of sources that don't help you become the best version of yourself or make you feel "less than." This exercise doesn't have to be just about removing sources of unhelpful information. You can add or follow new sources for education and inspiration, too. Just choose wisely.

Day 52

THE ONE THING THAT DETERMINES SUCCESS.

Real Life has a habit of behaving however it pleases. Any momentum you've established can come to an abrupt halt when Real Life shows up and shoves a crisis into your lap.

Your success, be it with a fitness regimen or any goal you have, will be determined by your ability to adapt to any given circumstance.

For example: Your habit is to work out four times a week. Then your boss gives you the biggest project of your life. Now you realistically have time for only two workouts, slashing in half your preferred routine. Will you adapt and say, "I can work with this! Two workouts may not be what I prefer, but it's all I can do right now, so I'll make the most of it while I focus on work"?

Or will you get discouraged and, rather than adapt and make do with what you have, stop working out completely until "things calm down at work," and lose all momentum in the process?

Health and fitness must be a lifetime endeavor, not a part-time hobby you pursue only when it's convenient and fits neatly into your schedule. This demands flexibility, a willingness to go with the flow.

Be malleable, like a sculptor's clay. Shape your plan to fit with your situation.

Forced to shorten your workout window? Adapt: Get in quality work with the time available by performing a few basic exercises and pushing each set harder than usual. Unable to prepare your usual meals, or find yourself in places with less-than-ideal food choices? Adapt: Make the best choices with what's available, or limit the quantity to a reasonable amount if you have no control over food quality. Did your gym close down? Adapt: Perform bodyweight workouts at home until you find a new place to join.

There will always be obstacles, and even setbacks. Become a Master Adapter. Start practicing now to cultivate the skill. It'll make your future challenges that much easier to overcome.

Think about a recent event that messed up your routine or posed a challenge. How could you have adapted to the situation? Or, perhaps, what do you need to adapt to right now?

Day 53
CHOOSE: EASY OR REWARDING.

Psychologist Albert Ellis said people often sacrifice long-term happiness because they're seduced by short-term, immediate pleasures.

The person trying to change her eating habits *wants* to improve her health, performance, and feel better (long-term happiness) but struggles to make the necessary choices to bring that outcome to fruition. She frequently turns to fast food and readily available high-calorie, low-nutrition foods (short-term pleasure).

The easy way is what comes natural to us, perhaps what we've always done. It usually provides instant gratification—no waiting for a long-term payoff. The rewarding way is, unfortunately, usually the difficult way, at least in the short term.

Skipping a workout because you "just don't feel like doing it" may be the easy way and instantly gratifying, but repeated long term, it's certainly not rewarding.

Trying new foods, attempting new recipes, and prepping a week's worth of lunches to take to work that will support the nutrition habits you're trying to build may be difficult initially, but the effort will be worth it because it will produce the long-term rewards you're after.

Sometimes an action can provide both instant and long-term rewards. For example, the person who skips after-work training sessions may have to exercise in the morning before work. The habit will provide long-term rewards and *immediate* benefits that come from the autonomous choice to do something good for her health.

Sometimes we do things because they're easiest in the moment, not realizing the difficult thing will lead to the desired rewards. There is good news: The more frequently you do the difficult, reward-producing things, the more ingrained they become, eventually requiring less conscious effort. They will be part of your lifestyle routine, just like showering, brushing your teeth, going to work, walking the dog, doing the dishes.

Do you frequently do the easy thing that provides immediate gratification? What hard(er) thing are you avoiding that's sacrificing the long-term results you desire?

Day 54
BE MORE.

Be more is a popular phrase that's been embraced by many as a lifestyle motto. It's even the cornerstone theme of the book *Lift Like a Girl: Be More, Not Less*.

The unfortunate truth about sayings like *be more* and the similar *become the best version of yourself* is that they've become a platitude. They're so common that they've lost their meaning.

There's no singular definition of what *be more* means or what it looks like when practiced. That's because it's up to each individual to define for herself what it means to *be more*.

In the arena of health and fitness, the *be more* mantra can mean choosing to use fitness to build up your strength, stamina, quality of life, and self-confidence instead of being solely about losing weight and looking better in clothes. It can also mean refusing to allow numbers (the scale, measurements, weight on the barbell, clothing size) and even the way you eat and move your body to define you or have any connotations about your self-worth.

Health and fitness should help you *be* and *become* the best version of yourself; it should build you up, not tear you down. What this looks like and how it's executed is up to you, and may even change over time.

Outside the gym, you choose what it means to *be more* according to the many roles you fulfill and the values you live by. You define it for yourself.

Today, how will you choose to be more?

Day 55
THINGS TO DO. THINGS NOT TO DO.

There's a symbiotic two-step process required to achieve what you don't currently have, to attain the results or an outcome you've never experienced.

Step 1: Do things you're not currently doing.

Step 2: Stop doing things you are currently doing.

There are instances where one step may conveniently replace the other. For example, stop skipping workouts (what you're currently doing) by scheduling them at a more convenient time, follow a program that's more enjoyable, set goals that ignite motivation, so the workouts are performed regularly (what you're not currently doing).

Other instances may take diligent and deliberate practice. Stop the verbal assaults that follow when you see your reflection in the mirror or look at yourself in photographs. Prepare ready-to-eat meals (or have the kitchen stocked) so that you have nourishing options after a long day and don't give in to visiting the drive through.

What are some things you currently do that you could stop doing that will help you achieve your goals?

What are some things you're currently not doing that you could?

Day 56
PARADOX, PART I.

The hedonist worldview advises you to seek pleasure above all else. You simply can't get enough of the good things life has to offer, so acquire as much pleasure as you can, while you have the privilege of being alive. Maybe you've known people who embrace that philosophy, but know it's not as pleasant as it's made out to be when that lifestyle catches up to them (or proves to be shallow and empty).

Then there's the paradoxical view one can take, especially with regards to food. The person who practices restraint and moderation, with calorie-dense not-super-nutritious foods, for example, actually enjoys them *more* than the person who consumes them in excess.

Restraint can provide a happy medium between the excessive swings of the pendulum from deprivation to decadence. Between being neurotic with food choices and inattentive.

The person who chooses to primarily eat nutrient-dense foods (lean proteins, whole grains, fruits and vegetables, nuts and seeds, fish, dairy, beans) and is selective about the tasty high-calorie, low-nutrient foods she eats (cakes, cookies, candy, ice cream, fried foods) will, in fact, enjoy those foods more.

She can turn down the offer of breakroom cookies without feeling deprived, because she instead plans to enjoy a slice of cheesecake that evening at her favorite restaurant.

She knows that what matters most for health is eating minimally-processed foods most often, and that it's important to enjoy favorite foods that don't fit that criteria without any guilt by eating them in moderate, less-frequent amounts.

By practicing restraint with all the tasty treats and convenience foods around her, and selectively choosing which ones she will enjoy in moderate amounts, she avoids the exhausting swings between depriving herself of enjoying her favorite foods and mindlessly indulging in them.

Is there a less-than-nutritious food you eat often? Could having it *less* often or in smaller amounts enhance the satisfaction you get from it?

Day 57
PARADOX, PART II.

Conversely, the other side of the hedonistic "seek out as much pleasure as possible" coin is the implication to actively avoid pain and discomfort.

Here we find one of the often unforeseen benefits of strength training and cardiovascular exercise. By intentionally exposing yourself to discomfort (lifting a heavy load multiple times, performing high-intensity intervals, maintaining steady-state activity for a 20-minute bout—you know, the uncomfortable stuff), not only is tolerance to the stimulus built, allowing you to do even more over time, but you discover that you're capable of enduring discomfort.

This means that when you face an unexpected situation where you must rely on your strength or endurance, you'll be more equipped to take on the challenge. The feeling of discomfort and strain won't be foreign to you; it'll be familiar, and far less daunting as a result.

The argument could also be made that frequent exposure to a challenging, even uncomfortable stimulus (like an intelligently designed strength training program and cardiovascular exercise regimen) makes relaxation more enjoyable and rewarding, too.

Think about it. Does a meal ever taste as good as it does when it satiates true hunger?

Do you appreciate a glass of ice water more than when it quenches thirst brought on by activity that left you parched and sweating?

And how about relaxation? Isn't it the most rewarding when it proceeds strenuous activity?

Simply trying to satisfy desires and seek pleasure while avoiding discomfort doesn't lead to enjoyment. The opposite is true:

Through restraint and deliberate selection, we enjoy our food more. Through repeated exercise, we become stronger and more resilient, have greater mental fortitude and endurance, and have a greater appreciation for relaxation.

How can you put this paradox to work for you?

Day 58

NOT ALWAYS ABOUT SAYING NO.

on't eat too many potato chips. Don't skip workouts. Don't needlessly chastise yourself.

With all the "don'ts" surrounding exercise and nutrition, it's easy to think a health and fitness lifestyle largely means saying "no." Turning down the tasty treats you're offered, even when it's a special occasion. Choosing not to eat fast food, even when you're too exhausted to shop and cook at home. Choosing not to skip your workout, even when plopping down on the couch after a stressful day sounds more enjoyable.

For many, saying "no" more often to dessert or a sugary beverage may be an important win, and a habit worth cultivating to improve their health and mental fitness. Others need to say "no" to the temptation to skip their workouts.

But some need to be able to say "yes" to their favorite dessert or fast food meal, and be able to enjoy it without being overcome with guilt or anxiety.

Some need to be able to say "yes" to taking a day off from the gym without any negative emotions clinging to that decision.

Health and fitness victories come in many forms. Some are physical, like performing a workout. Some are from choosing not to engage in an action, such as saying "no" to the breakroom potato chips or mindless snacking in front of the TV. Some are mental, like eating a couple cookies without a side order of guilt, or choosing to skip the gym because a family-time activity presented itself.

Don't become obsessed with saying "no" and "don't" on your journey. Remember, there are times when saying "yes" is the real victory.

Day 59
RENEW, RIGHT NOW.

As humans, we have a beautiful ability we take for granted. Often, we neglect it entirely.

What is it? The ability to renew our sense of self and purpose *at any moment*. It doesn't matter what you did five minutes ago; you can renew your concentration and focus this instant.

The past several months may have been the most challenging of your life, to the point you thought you may be crushed by the pressure. But you're here now, and in this moment, you can start fresh. Like putting a pen to a blank sheet of paper, you can start writing a new chapter. Right now, you can decide how to face today's challenges.

On a smaller, more manageable scale, you can choose to reject feeling guilty about missing a workout or not applying the nutrition habits you're trying to embrace. You can choose to view your upcoming workout as an opportunity to see what your body can do, instead of thinking about it as a chore or, worse, as punishment.

If you've gotten off track and skipped a few workouts, you can renew your focus and do a workout today, even if it's a 20-minute session. If your food choices haven't included mostly nutritious options, you can renew your commitment to self-care with the next meal or snack.

You have the power at every moment to renew your mindset. Embrace it.

If you're fortunate enough to be going through a wonderful time in your life, enjoy it. But keep this lesson in mind, so you will be better prepared when the next storm starts rolling in. The good times are great opportunities to prepare for future adversities.

Right now, do you need to renew your mindset? Because you can, this very instant.

Day 60

RIP IT OUT BY THE ROOTS.

How many of the following statements sound familiar?

- Exercise being an act of atonement for eating a not-super-healthy food.
- Exercise being currency to "earn" the right to eat a favorite food.
- Labeling certain foods and food groups "good" and others "bad."
- Feeling guilty after eating any food.
- Labeling parts of your body as "flaws."
- Berating yourself for slip-ups instead of responding with compassion.

All of these unhelpful ideas need to be extracted—ripped out, roots and all.

We weren't born with these thoughts imprinted in our minds. We learned them. Maybe you heard a friend rave about the grueling workout she did because she needed to "earn the right" to eat a cheeseburger. Maybe as a child you heard a female relative say, "I've been so good with my diet, I deserve to cheat!" to justify eating well beyond the point of satiety. Maybe your social group echoes similar comments, too.

These experiences can plant seeds in our mind, and the more we hear them, and then start to *embrace* them for ourselves, those seeds sprout and grow roots. The more we repeat these mantras or are exposed to them, the roots penetrate deeper, making them tougher to remove.

This is why certain habits we want to change can be extremely challenging to break. Their roots have grown thick and are buried deep. They can't simply be plucked out. They must be excavated.

It's worth the effort, removing those unhealthy perceptions about food, working out, and our bodies. Be patient and persistent, and know that you may have to shovel mounds of dirt before the roots are exposed, allowing you to remove them completely.

What ideas or thoughts do you need to rip out by the roots? More importantly, what exactly will you start doing differently to make it happen?

Days 61-70

Day 61
WHAT IF THIS HAPPENED TO A FRIEND?

"I am my own worst critic," we proudly declare. While this commitment to self-awareness can be tremendously useful, when applied correctly, it can also be a tool of destruction, especially when applied to situations involving food and fitness.

If you were to "blow your diet" for a couple weeks and gain a few pounds, how would you respond? You may harshly berate yourself, chastising your lack of self-control. Maybe you'd even emotionally beat yourself up and call yourself a failure. Being your own worst critic in this manner is not helpful.

In times when you choose self-flagellation as a response, a practical and helpful psychological exercise is to use projective visualization. Rather than responding to *your* behavior, act as though you were talking to a friend, or even to a child, who had the experience and was asking for your advice on how to respond.

It's unlikely you'd recommend a response defined by self-loathing, guilt, and harsh criticism. No, you'd see the situation for what it truly is: *not a big deal*. So don't treat it like one in your own experience.

You know, for example, that bringing lunch to work helps prevent you from giving in to fast food temptation, which typically leads to less-than-ideal choices in the days that follow. But maybe one day you forget your lunch, or just didn't feel like making it the night before, and wound up getting food from the drive through and then used that experience to justify a lack of healthful food choices for a few days. Instead of beating yourself up, tell yourself exactly what you'd say if this same thing happened to a friend. Maybe, "If something can be gleaned from the slip-up to help prevent it from happening in the future, that's terrific. Otherwise, don't be upset about something that can't be changed. Harsh criticism isn't productive. The best thing to do is move forward, unburdened from unnecessary guilt."

Don't "move forward" in an obsessive or punishing way, but in a *"What happened happened, it's over with, and I will get back on track"* way. The healthy approach is to learn from the experience and use that knowledge to prepare for a similar situation in the future, so you can handle it more productively.

Think about a recent event when you tore into yourself with extreme criticism. Then ask yourself, "How would I tell a friend to respond if this happened to them?"

When you find yourself in such a situation in the future, recall this exercise and put it to use. Remove yourself from the experience and view it like it happened to a friend or loved one and use that imagery to guide your response.

Day 62
BETTER, OR TIRED?

It's currently popular for people to showcase their "brutal" workouts on social media. Images of people collapsed on the floor, "sweat angels" lingering on the gym mat after the workout, and hovering over a trash can to highlight their workout intensity.

Such images might get likes and comments, but exhausting yourself, brutal soreness, or teetering on the brink of vomiting are not accurate indicators to gauge the effectiveness of a workout.

Don't get caught in the trap of equating exhaustion and a sweat-drenched t-shirt with having performed a good workout. Getting better—improving performance over time (not necessarily every workout or even every week)—is what matters most. And you needn't get brutally sore or exhausted regularly to make that happen.

Make your exercise technique more efficient; perform an extra rep than last time; perform an extra set; increase the weight; cover a greater distance in the same time period; just *get in the work* even if you know it's not going to be a great workout (these workouts count too, because they help the roots of the workout habit grow deeper and help you accept the fact that not every workout is going to be awesome, nor do they have to be—the goal is to do your best on any given day).

Don't chase soreness or exhaustion. These are poor markers that have no positive influence on the effectiveness of a workout. Get better, gradually, over time. And, of course, *have fun*.

Have you been trapped in the mindset of thinking you must finish each workout utterly exhausted, or that you must feel sore the next day? How can you start breaking free from this fallacy with your next workout? Or, simply, how can you focus solely on doing a little better than last time?

Day 63

DON'T GIVE FEAR THE REINS.

"Fear cuts deeper than swords," the young Arya Stark repeats throughout the book *A Game of Thrones*. The lesson, taught by her sword instructor, became her mantra. When faced with frightful situations, even the looming possibility of her own death, she clung to the words "fear cuts deeper than swords" to prevent fear from paralyzing her and dictating her choices.

We can confidently rule out the possibility of being caught in a sword fight in our lives (thankfully), but we allow fear to restrain us in other, often unnoticed, ways.

Countless women allow the fear of "looking silly" to keep them from strength training. Some allow the fear of failing to prevent them from making changes to their eating habits. Others allow the fear of not being the best to hold them back from participation.

Giving fear the reins to determine how you will live your life is more dangerous, and harmful, than any likely less-than-desirable outcome. When fear is allowed to be the decision maker, we may *think* we're making the safer choice, but what we're really doing is becoming passengers in our journey. More bluntly, we become a slave to fear.

When you choose to face fear and refuse to relinquish control to it, you discover what you're capable of doing and withstanding. Oftentimes you'll realize, "I was worried about *that*? That wasn't that bad at all!"

The next time fear seizes your mind, telling you not to go to that part of the gym, not to participate in a certain activity, not to attempt building new habits, or anything else out of fear of looking silly or not doing as well as others, cast it aside. Don't give in to it.

How else will you know what you're capable of doing unless you get out of your comfort zone? How many enjoyable memories will you miss out on, until you refuse to let fear paralyze you?

Day 64
NOT GOOD. NOT BAD.

"For there is nothing either good or bad, but thinking makes it so."

These wise words are one of the most memorable quotations in Shakespeare's *Hamlet*. That saying *sounds* nice, and it's experienced a resurgence thanks to the growing popularity of Stoic ideology. Sadly, though, it's turning into an inane platitude, as is the fate of many great sayings.

It would be a mistake to underestimate the immense power of that sentence and its many variations. (Another popular version comes from Epictetus: "People are not disturbed by things, but the views they take of them.") No matter how you express it, it's an idea that can put tremendous power in your hands when you choose to live by it.

Here's an example you may be able to relate to: You go on a diet and follow it without deviation for a month. Then the temptation of your favorite dessert beckons, and you give in. With that one dessert you proclaim to have "blown your diet." Then you feel guilty for not being able to "stick to the plan." You screwed up and continue to mentally berate yourself.

You're not upset because you ate dessert. You're upset because you're assigning a judgment to that event. You are *choosing* to label it a screw-up.

Eating your favorite dessert or fast food meal is not bad. Missing a workout isn't bad. Making a string of less-than-ideal food choices isn't bad. Succumbing to deeply ingrained old habits you're trying to break isn't bad.

Stop berating yourself for things not worthy of punishment. Stop sticking "good" and "bad" labels to elements of what is supposed to be a health and fitness lifestyle. You have the power to choose how you view and respond to situations. Commit to doing so in a helpful, productive way.

What events (eating sweets, missing a workout, gaining a few pounds) do you label as "bad"? Be mindful of your response to such instances. Remember, you choose what they mean. Use that power for good.

Day 65
I'LL GET STARTED WHEN …

Ever notice how we attempt to justify our procrastination in breaking a habit or forming a new one, or restarting our plan after a slip-up or setback?

"I'll start my new diet on Monday," you may say the Friday before, then use that erroneous logic to eat with reckless abandon all weekend. You're going to "get back on track" Monday, so why not cut loose in the meantime?

"I'll start over next week," you may say after missing a scheduled workout during the middle of the week. Rather than perform the workout later that day or the next, the missed workout is used as an excuse to take the rest of the week off to "start fresh" Monday.

"I'll start on New Year's Day."

"I'll start once things calm down at work."

"I'll start when the kids go back to school."

"I'll start once the holidays are over."

"I'll start when I have more energy."

"I'll start when I feel motivated."

"I'll start when this lingering injury goes away."

How many of those statements have you made?

There can always be numerous excuses to put something off, to restart at a more convenient time, to feel discouraged and choose to quit, to procrastinate because who chooses to get back to working out or making nutrient-dense food choices on a Tuesday?

When we realize we're feeding ourselves weak justifications, and force ourselves to stare the truth in the face, then we're free to realize there is no good choice other than starting (or restarting) *now*. Today. The first step doesn't even have to be big. It can be an action as simple as including a salad or vegetable with your next meal, or going for a 15-minute walk after work.

Do *something*, and do it immediately.

Is there something you need, or want, to do that you've been putting off?

Day 66
KNOW WHEN TO COAST.

One of the worst assumptions to be made with a health and fitness routine is the need to go "all in," all the time. If we're not striving to perform every workout, flawlessly, and to make the best choices at every meal, then we think we're failing.

There's an appropriate time to put in extra effort, to be more diligent with food choices and workouts to get further ahead. If, for example, life is less hectic during a certain time of year, like when the kids go back to school, then by all means seize that opportunity to dedicate more time and attention to workouts and eating habits. Use that time to your advantage to take a greater leap forward to your goals. Take that opportunity to make more progress in a shorter time period while you have the luxury of doing so.

The same mentality applies to occasions when devoting ample time to fitness is not an option, when time is not a luxury and you can only carve out enough to do the minimum. This is okay too, and can even be the smart decision. Rather than the usual one-hour workouts, perform 30-minute workouts. Work hard and do your best in that time, then get out of the gym and on with the rest of your life.

It's okay to coast, to do the minimum. This way you retain the results and progress you've made while continuing to practice the workout habit, but without having to devote an immense amount of effort, or time. (The good news is that research has demonstrated that strength and muscle can be maintained by reducing workout volume to one third of previous workout program levels.)[2]

Know when to coast and adjust your regimen as needed. When

---

[2]. L.D. Tavares, E.O. de Souza, C. Ugrinowitsch, G.C. Laurentino, H. Roschel, A.Y. Aihara, F.N. Cardoso, and V. Tricoli, "Effects of Different Strength Training Frequencies During Reduced Training Period on Strength and Muscle Cross-Sectional Area," Eur J Sport Sci (July 2017), https://ncbi.nlm.nih.gov/pubmed/28316261.

other priorities arise, life stress increases noticeably, or you just need a bit of a break from dedicating a lot of time and energy on training, perform abbreviated workouts or commit to doing three 30-minute workouts per week. Just find a way coast through the chaos.

Day 67
DON'T COMPLAIN.

We complain about our weight.
We complain about our cellulite.
We complain about having to work out.
We complain about needing to eat more protein and fiber.
We complain about not being as strong or fit as we think we should be.
We complain about having to be selective with the not-super-healthy foods we eat.

But does complaining ever make you feel better? Does it ever change anything?

Complaining is merely an act of indulging our emotions. Things didn't go the way you wanted them to or you don't see results as quickly as you desired, so you gripe, moan, and occasionally give in to self-pity.

If something needs to change to make the process easier or more enjoyable, change it.

Maybe you're complaining about your workouts because you don't enjoy them and you're following a plan out of what feels like an obligation. Do something different. Set goals that ignite motivation, or at least reduce dread. Use the equipment and exercises you prefer with strength training, for example.

If you're following an overly restrictive diet that you know isn't practical long term and you're always complaining about it, change it.

Make the process as simple and enjoyable as possible. Do what you need to do, and when you catch yourself on the verge of complaining, stop. Remind yourself that it doesn't help. It won't make that workout any easier, or make your thighs slim down any quicker, or help you add more weight to the barbell any sooner.

If you discover your workout routine needs to change, you need to simplify your nutrition habits or make some other modification, do it. If what you've been doing isn't working, troubleshoot. Look back at exactly what you did (or maybe didn't do), reassess the approach, and take action that will lead you in the direction you want to go.

But don't waste time complaining, because it won't help.

Day 68

HOME IN ON WHAT MATTERS.

Life is short.
Even if you live to the remarkable age of 110, your life would still be short.

When put in the context of the thousands of years of recorded human history that preceded your birth, the billions of people swallowed up by time, and the thousands of years that will proceed your departure from this world, you can clearly see how brief your time here is.

Thinking about how one hundred years is a fleeting instant in the vast span of time shouldn't be scary. It should help you see how silly it is to get upset over a lackluster workout, a week of overindulging, a month of skipped workouts, a ten-pound weight gain, not setting a personal record you'd been chasing, or an injury you must work around while you heal.

This isn't an excuse to use the *you-only-live-once* attitude to live recklessly and not invest in self-care because we're all going to die. The understanding of how short our time here is should help you home in on what truly matters, and realize how much time we spend on the myriad that doesn't.

Life is short. Use that lens to clearly identify what's most important to you. Who you want to be, today, and the person you want to become while you have the chance. To properly put in perspective the events we catastrophize unnecessarily.

Missed the last few scheduled workouts? No big deal. You're one workout away from getting back on track. You can do it today.

Not making the most healthful food choices lately? That's not something to punish yourself over. You're one meal away from getting back on track.

Struggling to appreciate your body for what it can do? Make that the focus of the next workout.

Frustrated with an injury that's preventing you from exercising the way you prefer? There's still plenty you *can* do, and that is where your effort should go.

Life is short. It would behoove you to not let the insignificant things (which, quite often, are disguised as "big" things until we stop and analyze what they truly are) rob you of your time (your one true commodity) and mental energy. When you find yourself getting upset over anything pertaining to food and fitness, put it into context. Then get back on track.

Day 69

A WHAT-IF EXERCISE.

Imagine this:

For the past two months you've performed three strength training workouts every week. You're getting stronger, you feel incredible, and you're noticing changes to your body. Finally, you're hitting your stride and momentum is accumulating.

But today, you trip walking down the stairs and break your ankle. You'll be in a cast for six weeks and can't put any weight on that leg. What will you do?

"I just *knew* something would happen to screw up my progress!" you could respond. You could compound the frustration of the injury and choose to stop going to the gym until you're fully recovered and make less-than-ideal food choices too because, what's the point in eating well if you can't even work out?

You could choose to immediately take stock of all the activities and exercises you can't do and feel sorry for yourself. Or instead, you could focus exclusively on the many activities you *can* do.

Your upper body isn't affected by the incident. While you may have to use different equipment than you normally prefer to work out with, you can still make excellent progress in other ways. In fact, you can make better progress than ever in certain areas or exercises than you otherwise would, since those areas/exercises will now receive more attention. Meanwhile, your uninjured leg can still be trained in many ways; research has demonstrated that the non-trained limb can receive some benefits from training the fully-functioning limb.[3]

---

3. Justin W. Andrushko, Joel L. Lanovaz, Kelsey M. Bjorkman, Saija A. Kontulainen, and Jonathan P. Farthing, "Unilateral Strength Training Leads to Muscle-Specific Sparing Effects During Opposite Homologous Limb Immobilization," Journal of Applied Physiology (April 2018), https://physiology.org/doi/full/10.1152/japplphysiol.00971.2017.

You can turn what initially appeared to be a disadvantage into an advantage, or at least an opportunity rather than a setback.

Practice this theoretical what-if exercise regularly and keep its lessons close at hand because, at some point, fortune will put your resolve to the test. Hopefully it won't be as drastic as a broken bone, but by mentally preparing for it, you (a) won't be as shocked by the experience and (b) you'll immediately know how to pragmatically respond.

Day 70
GREAT LEARNING OPPORTUNITIES.

When was the last time you ate so much delicious food that you were uncomfortably full? How about instead of enjoying one piece of cake, did you have two? Did you eat the entire container of something, instead of the reasonable quantity you intended?

If you were on a diet during that incident, or trying to forge sustainable health-promoting eating habits, these instances might be labeled as mistakes. You overate. You ate too much cake. You did not eat in moderation.

And then what happened? If you're like a lot of women on this journey, you focused on the *mistakes* themselves. "I shouldn't have eaten so much …"

Instead of obsessing over the mistakes themselves, focus on how you can *learn* from them. Why did you overeat? Did you skip a meal earlier in the day, or was there an emotional trigger that led you to comfort yourself with food? Did you eat directly out of a container instead of getting a serving and putting the rest away?

Mistakes can be excellent learning opportunities. But you must first calm down, accept what happened, look at the event objectively and ask, "Why did I do this?" Then use that knowledge going forward. Don't panic from overeating and then obsess over how to "undo" the damage by limiting your food intake the next day or performing an extra workout. As you know by now, that punishment mentality will not help you.

Identify the triggers or circumstances that cause you to overeat or feel like you lose control, especially for instances that have a repeating pattern. (Overeating is something everyone does on occasion and is not worth getting upset over or labeling a "mistake.") Common triggers can be emotional eating, eating food directly from containers, waiting until you're ravenous to eat, or not having healthful options in the house. Whatever the catalyst might be, you can train yourself to identify it in the future, so you can extinguish the tiny flame and prevent it from turning into a raging fire that's more difficult to put out.

Days 71-80

Day 71

CALL OUT THE NONSENSE.

Self-compassion is a skill worth cultivating, especially if you're accustomed to chastising yourself harshly for slip-ups or even flat-out failures. You can't build yourself up if you're always tearing yourself back down.

Another useful skill that intertwines with self-compassion is practicing pragmatic objectivity. In other words, develop the ability to call out your own bullshit.

Sometimes, in order to reach your goals or to finally start your journey, what you really need is candid honesty. You missed the last three strength training workouts? You can skip the useless atonement and respond with self-compassion and understanding, but don't delude yourself, either.

Did you skip your workouts just because you didn't "feel like" doing them, or because you wanted to watch your favorite Netflix show? Call yourself out.

Are you not implementing your desired nutrition changes because fast food is easier than taking your lunch to work, or because you don't have your kitchen stocked with healthful options? Call yourself out.

Is your mindset not changing as quickly as you'd like because you're not really doing the work to make that happen, like journaling and being mindful of your self-talk throughout the day? Call yourself out.

Sometimes extenuating circumstances take priority over a workout, meal-prepping session, or journaling. But sometimes the real culprit is wallowing in your own delusions and excuses. In those times, you need to hold yourself accountable for your lack of progress.

When and where are you making excuses? Where are you *truly* not putting in the effort, while trying to convince yourself that you have been?

You can have self-compassion for your errors and learn from them. At the same time, you can also expunge the nonsense. Call yourself out when needed to clearly reveal what you're doing, what you're not doing, and what you need to start doing today.

Day 72

WHEN "GOOD" BEATS "BEST."

What you can do *consistently* long term will always outperform what is "best," especially if the "best" option isn't practical or enjoyable.

You're told you must strength train three times per week if you want to achieve the best results possible. Perhaps your life is busier than ever and you can only realistically dedicate twice-weekly visits to the gym.

"If I can't do what's 'best,' what's the point in doing anything at all?" is a common response to such a situation.

Performing two workouts per week still provides numerous benefits, especially if you do it for months and years in succession. Sure, three may be a bit better than two for building strength and muscle, but two is unquestionably better than zero.

When chaos ensues, or you're experiencing elevated levels of stress, or you just want to do the bare minimum while focusing on other activities or interests, always remember that *good* can be good enough.

Aim for consistent progress over perfection.

Don't be blinded by overzealous comments that you must go "all in" to get results or that you must "fully commit" or relentlessly seek the "best" program, diet, whatever. There are options between nothing and (theoretical) perfection. Embrace that fact and make the most of what you can give, when you can give it.

Taking action, consistently, over the long term, is what produces results. So what if you achieve them a little slower? When you revolve your life around a routine that isn't doable for you, it only ends with you losing everything you achieved. Better to acquire results at a steadier pace and be able to maintain them (while also maintaining your sanity).

Day 73
YES YOU CAN HANDLE IT.

The poet Johann Wolfgang von Goethe said, "It is a great error to take oneself for more than is, or for less than one is worth."

You're probably aware of the dangers of being overly confident. Listening too much to your ego typically ends with learning an important lesson of humility. But how rarely do you contemplate the second part of Goethe's phrase? It is a disservice we do to ourselves to value ourselves at less than our true worth.

The intimidation or unfamiliarity of a situation might make you hesitate to act. Something you never anticipated shakes you to the core with its unwelcome arrival. It appears daunting, too cumbersome, so you utter "I can't handle this" as you retreat in defeat.

But underestimating yourself is not without consequences.

You are stronger, more capable, more resilient, more adaptable than you realize or give yourself credit for. Not realizing that can hold you back and hinder your growth.

Think about an event you were forced to face, one that you couldn't escape. Perhaps someone close to you died, a loved one was living with an illness, you lost your job unexpectedly, or you were the recipient of unsavory news. If someone asked you if you could overcome that challenge prior to it happening, you may have said "Absolutely not."

But you did overcome it. It didn't destroy you or crush you.

You're stronger than you realized back then. More resilient than you gave yourself credit for. You have the necessary tools within yourself to face life's challenges.

Don't undervalue yourself or your abilities.

Day 74
YOU DON'T HAVE TO HEALTH-IFY EVERYTHING.

There's a growing trend that encourages morphing every food into a healthier, "guiltless" version. To be certain, there's nothing wrong with modifying certain foods you eat regularly, like choosing to make oven-baked fries instead of the deep-fried variety if you eat them several times per week.

But the incessant need to make a healthier version, especially for foods only eaten occasionally, is absurd. Partly because these "healthier" versions often have the same number of calories as the food they're attempting to mimic, but mostly because of how this mindset can exacerbate a fear of food. People see their favorite foods and their instinct is, "I can't eat this unless I make it healthier."

Think of a family-favorite food that you enjoy on a certain holiday. Maybe it's a homemade cheesecake, for example. If you've recently come to believe every decadent dessert must receive a healthy makeover and replace the all-time favorite recipe with a "healthier" one, the likelihood is that you and your family will be immensely disappointed with the result. What, then, was the purpose of making the "healthier" version? Other than saving a few calories (maybe) on a food you didn't enjoy, nothing was achieved.

The better option would have been to make the original, favorite, only-eaten-on-occasion dessert, *enjoy a reasonable amount*, then move on.

Choose your battles. Aim to eat mostly minimally-processed foods, get sufficient protein and fiber, and eat plenty of vegetables on a regular basis. Then enjoy the not-super-healthy foods you love most on occasion, in moderate amounts, absolutely guilt free. (As a reminder, every food should be eaten guilt free.)

There's nothing wrong with experimenting with healthier

versions of your favorite foods and swapping them out for lower-calorie or more healthful options. But don't feel obligated to do it with everything, especially if it produces an inferior result you don't enjoy.

Food should not be feared; it should be enjoyed. Some things we should simply eat more often, and others less often. You can find this balance when you systematically remove the fear and emotion that has been tied to what you eat.

Day 75
WHEN WHAT YOU FEEL DOESN'T COINCIDE WITH WHAT YOU SEE.

It's the same story, echoed by a multitude of women. Their workouts leave them feeling great. They feel strong, energized, proud of themselves for what they accomplished and the progress revealed in their training logs. However, that satisfaction turns to disappointment when the reflection in the mirror or photos of themselves don't parallel that feeling.

When how you feel and how you think you look seem to be at odds, the result is frustration. What can you do about it? You have two options.

Option 1: Focus on feeding the feelings of strength, accomplishment, and empowerment, since you can experience these daily. Focus on collecting those wins each day, and you'll get closer and closer to the outcome you want.

For example, when your workout is done, look back at what you did.

"I squatted five more pounds today."

"I got out of my comfort zone and finally went into the free-weight area of the gym."

"I took extra time to learn how to correctly perform an exercise, and I'm confident doing it now."

"I was able to use a higher resistance level for my cardio."

"I didn't feel as strong today so I used the workout as an opportunity to hone exercise technique with lighter weights."

Focus on what you accomplish via your actions and self-talk.

Option 2: Think of your fitness journey as a trip across the country. You're currently at Point A, and you want to get to Point B. Only in this situation, you may not be able to get there on a non-stop private jet. The pace will be slower. You may even have to walk at some point. But there will be much to be enjoyed along the way if you take the time to look around and embrace the experience.

You may not arrive at the destination with haste, but you can get there. Even better, you can enjoy the journey.

Day 76
CUT CONVERSATIONS SHORT.

Have you ever noticed how quickly a thought like "I can't believe I ate all that food" can escalate into a lengthy mental conversation that concludes with you feeling terrible about yourself?

"Why did I eat so much? I feel fat and gross."

"I shouldn't have eaten so much—I overdid it. This is a setback."

"I knew I'd screw up again. I always do this!"

"Maybe I should try to undo the damage."

A goal worth striving for isn't necessarily to *prevent* such conversations, but to realize that you can cut them short. Giving in to that first thought just allows it to escalate and grow. When you catch yourself criticizing a choice you would have rather not made, or wishing you had taken some other action, stop it. Immediately. Don't allow the initial thought to spiral into a negative self-talk tirade.

You can say, "You know what? I'm not going to play this game. I'm not going to turn this into something."

We can't always stop ourselves from getting upset or disappointed with our choices—that initial reflexive response is difficult to prevent—but we can cut the conversations short and refuse to allow them to intensify. Remember that next time you're criticizing yourself.

Day 77
SEE PAST THE FAÇADE.

The health and wellness market is a multi-billion dollar industry. Within that industry is an abundance of misinformation, sham products, and schemes disguised as health-promoting, life-changing solutions.

Obsessive eating habits are masked as "dedication"; performing a grueling workout for overindulging is disguised as "discipline"; narcissism is considered "inspiring" or "influential"; questionable and unregulated supplements that lack evidence for the beneficial effects they claim to produce are shamelessly peddled.

Don't let the façade fool you. Look behind it and see what is *really* there.

Sometimes it's clever marketing tactics tempting you to open your wallet by poking your insecurities. Sometimes it's tribalism pitched by a person deeply convinced that their way to health and fitness is *the way* for everyone. Sometimes it's just vanity, greed, ignorance.

Beware of sources trying to sell you happiness and beauty when they don't put forth viable evidence, but instead use ear-grabbing terminology and sensationalized promises. If you look carefully, it's apparent that they're more interested in receiving attention than helping people.

Remember, the foundation of what should define a healthy lifestyle has already been proven: frequent exercise, eating mostly minimally-processed foods (including sufficient protein, fiber, fruits and vegetables); getting adequate sleep, managing stress, not smoking or doing drugs, and limiting alcohol consumption. None of these things are exciting, sexy, new, or groundbreaking—that's why they're often dismissed.

The details and execution of the variables like nutrition and exercise should be tailored to your preferences and lifestyle to ensure adherence, and the finer details may evolve as research advances, but those basics are unlikely to waver.

There are no shortcuts. No magical pills, drinks, powders, or programs. No viable "one weird trick." Once you truly embrace that fact, seeing past the façade becomes much easier. You can look beyond what they *want you to see* and you can identify what is really there.

What façade has distracted you from doing what matters most?

Day 78
NOT MISSED, UNTIL IT'S GONE.

When prompted with the question, "If you could change anything about your body, what would it be?" you likely have a string of answers ready: your weight, body shape, hair color, stretch marks, bra size, height, maybe physical strength and stamina.

Here's a better question: What physical ability would you miss if it was abruptly taken from you?

In a world that's smothering us with a relentless pursuit of self-improvement, we think if we're not constantly improving that we must be failing. So we pursue More, Better, Newer, Upgraded. With health and fitness this can also mean Leaner, Smaller, Fitter, Stronger, Curvier.

Most of us are so busy chasing improvement that we neglect, or at the very least fail to appreciate, what we've already achieved and the abilities we possess.

Think about it again: What ability would you miss if it was suddenly taken from you?

The ability to hold this book in your hands and read?

Being able to walk?

Preparing a meal?

Playing with your children?

Going to the gym for a workout?

It's so easy to take for granted the incredible things your body can do. This is especially true in difficult times, or when you're facing injury or illness. There are things you likely take for granted (as we all do), things you wouldn't miss until the instant something threatened to take them from you.

This is a psychology technique known as negative visualization—contemplating what you have, what you can do, then imagining your life without them—and it can be a powerful tool.

Reframe what you value. Look at, and appreciate, what you would miss. After all, there's no guarantee these abilities will always be yours to enjoy.

Then go do something with those abilities.

Day 79

MUSTER UP SOME GRIT.

Abby Wambach, two-time Olympic gold medalist and FIFA Women's World Cup champion, had countless remarkable moments in her soccer career.

One in particular, however, had nothing to do with head butting the ball into the back of the net or assisting a teammate with a game-winning goal. A mid-air collision with an opponent sent her to the ground, with blood pouring from a gash on her forehead. As she was lying on the ground, blood running down her face and pooling on the turf, it was easy to think her playing time in that game was done.

But Abby wasn't done. She went to the sideline, *got the gaping head wound stapled shut*, and went back on the field to play.

Yet when you miss a few workouts, eat fried foods with reckless abandon for a weekend, or berate yourself with negative self-talk after stepping on the bathroom scale, how easy is it for you to want to give up? You profess to have "screwed up" yet again, or decide that this entire process is too hard, or the results are coming too slowly, and consider quitting entirely. But there's no real "wound" in these scenarios. You're simply *choosing* to *create* one and use it as an excuse to quit or chastise yourself.

What if you had a bit more grit? What if, instead of wasting even a single moment thinking about quitting or complaining, you immediately sought to stop the bleeding and got back into the thick of the action, ready to try again?

Obstacles will always appear. Setbacks are inevitable, and some will keep you down longer than others. Some may simply shock you in the moment, and others will draw blood; neither has to stop you.

There's time left on the clock. You just need to muster up the grit to keep going.

Day 80
DO THE OPPOSITE.

Most women have been on a diet. Most women have been on *numerous* diets, in fact, with the sole goal of losing weight. And most women, unfortunately, have been led to believe that dieting, trying to get skinny, or hating parts of their body is simply part of what it means to be a woman.

We talk to our friends about hating our thighs, our cellulite, our tummy or back bulges, our short or long legs. Then we talk about how we "have to go to the gym" to "fix" these parts of our bodies all while discussing the next diet we plan on trying.

All of this is ridiculous, and we need to stop taking part in it.

It's time to do the opposite of what you've been conditioned to believe is the only food and fitness path for a woman.

Forget about burning calories or "fixing" a part of your body with exercise. Choose to work out to get stronger. To feel incredible. To manage stress and invest in self-care.

Learn to embrace and love words like *muscle, strength* and *endurance*. Muscle is beautiful, and strength and endurance are empowering.

Don't obsess over the foods you "shouldn't" eat. Choose instead to focus on eating more nutrient-dense foods you enjoy.

Don't fear any food. Make room for your favorite foods in your eating habits and enjoy them occasionally in a moderate amount.

Don't fear setbacks or even outright failures. These are not definitive events; they can be incredible opportunities to expand your knowledge base, showing you what wasn't working so you can more easily figure out what will.

Don't allow your happiness to hinge on attaining a certain bodyweight or shape or size or performance standard. Instead, choose to make *the process* as enjoyable as possible, so eating well and moving your body is something you *want to do* and *get to do*, not a chore you feel obligated to do.

Most importantly, create food and fitness habits that build you up, and reject those that attempt to tear you down.

How can you start taking this empowering, opposite approach with your food and fitness choices? Or, in what ways *have you been* practicing this over the past several weeks and what have been some of the results?

Days 81-90

Day 81
LOOK, THEN LAUGH.

You thought today was the day you'd set that personal record you'd been chasing. You felt incredible, had a great night's sleep, and all signs of the previous weeks' training indicated the record would happen today.

But it didn't. In fact, you didn't even get close to it.

Instantly you feel frustrated, then upset. You've been busting your butt for months to nail this goal. The more you think about all the time and effort you've exerted, the more annoyed you become.

Should this *really* be something that upsets you?

You could choose instead to stop, assess what happened, and laugh it off. "Well, that did *not* go as I expected!" Shrug it off with a laugh, then move on.

The failed personal record doesn't negate all the work you've done up to that point. The previous workouts still made you better, stronger, healthier, and further solidified the workout habit. So you didn't set your intended record today—so what? Maybe it was just an "off" day, maybe you underestimated the additional life stress that's been accumulating, maybe your workout program needs to be adjusted.

As another example, perhaps you were craving your favorite candy bar, but you ate yogurt with mixed berries instead to curb your appetite. A couple hours later, you still wanted that candy bar, but you ate something "healthy" instead, then snacked on other foods. Before you know it, you've eaten more calories than you would have consumed if you just enjoyed the candy bar you wanted. Instead of getting upset, you could laugh it off: "Guess I should've just had the candy bar—I would've been satisfied instead of eating a bunch of other stuff in its place!"

We are quick to take this food and fitness stuff too seriously, and judge ourselves too harshly. Sometimes the best thing you can do is just look at the situation you find yourself in, and laugh about it.

Day 82
YOU CAN'T ALTER THE PAST.

Improving your health and level of fitness, when distilled to its basic elements, is about eating nutritious foods *most of the time* and moving your body frequently and consistently.

But when you look at your own life, you know it is not quite that easy.

You already know what you *should* do when it comes to eating and moving your body. It's the consistent *execution* that can be the challenge.

Why is that?

It starts with your past. We've each had unique experiences in how we were raised, the foods we ate as children, the way our parents viewed physical activity, and how those lessons were taught to us (intentionally or otherwise). How we saw the women and men in our lives talk about their bodies and weight, and how their clothes fit. Whether we ate homemade meals at the table as a family, or everyone was in front of the TV with a fast food meal.

All these things shaped your perception of food, fitness, and body image. And you carry those perceptions with you into adulthood, for better or worse.

There's a lot to unravel when it comes to understanding why you view things the way you do. This is why health and fitness guidelines can't always be executed seamlessly with ease.

Your past cannot be changed. Sure, it might have been great if things were different. But they weren't. Even if you had great advantages and were raised in a family that prioritized nutritious foods and physical activity, you might still have gone off track and ended up with a mindset that doesn't serve you, like obsessive eating habits or a negative self-image.

Regardless of your history and any advantages or disadvantages it provided, you can choose *today* the actions you will take. Learn valuable lessons from your past if possible, but don't allow it to define who you will be today. Choose that for yourself.

You can always construct a new lifestyle, or simply make a few tweaks to improve it.

Day 83
"FEELING LIKE IT" ISN'T A REQUIREMENT.

If you always "felt like" doing a workout or choosing to eat a nutritious whole-food meal instead of a tasty deep-fried delicacy, then you'd have a much easier time achieving your health and fitness goals.

That isn't always the case.

You will not always *feel like* working out.

You will not always *feel like* eating vegetables.

You will not always *feel like* being mindful of what you tell yourself about the number on the bathroom scale or tape measure.

Thankfully, *feeling like* doing the actions that create your desired lifestyle and lead to the outcomes you want is not a requirement for doing the things that need to be done.

Feeling like doing good-for-you things is a nice bonus, but it's completely optional.

You don't always *feel like* going to work, but you go.

You don't always *feel like* brushing your teeth, but you do it.

You've never *felt like* filing your taxes, but you get it done.

You certainly have never *felt like* cleaning up pet vomit, but you do it.

Approach your workouts and nutrition habits in the same way—they are part of your life, and even though you won't always *feel like* doing these things, you will do them anyway. Not for punishment, or fear of losing results you've already achieved, or to attain the fickle and transient status quo, but because you're invested in self-care. Because you know it's crucial to keep the flame of habit flickering so it doesn't get extinguished.

Next time you catch yourself grumbling "I don't feel like working out today," quickly remind yourself, you don't need to feel like doing it to get it done.

Day 84
EXPECTATION BIAS.

Your thoughts and expectations can affect your experience.

If you *expect* to have a terrible workout from a bad night's sleep, you just might.

If you *expect* an expensive pre-workout supplement to drastically improve your workout performance, it very well may.

Likewise, if you become reliant on a pre-workout supplement and say you "can't work out without it" and suddenly have to, you may go into that workout expecting to underperform, and you just might.

If you *expect* a nagging ache to keep you out of the gym or away from your usual routine for a long period of time, it just might.

If you *expect* your menstrual cycle to have a negative effect on your workout performance, it very well may.

If you *expect* to have the ability to get stronger, faster, more conditioned, better coordinated, it's more likely to happen.

Our minds are powerful, and research has shown this to be the case with placebo and nocebo effects (experiencing positive or negative effects from an inert substance, respectively).[4] This isn't to say you can always think your way out of a bad workout or think your way to rapid results, but you should always be mindful of your thoughts and how they color your experiences.

Don't catastrophize a less-than-ideal situation by responding with frustration and grief—that will only compound its (possible) effects. Bad night's sleep? Don't assume you'll have a bad workout. Just go into it like you normally would and see how it goes. Adjust if needed, based on feedback from warm-up sets.

---

4. Hurst P., Schipof-Godart L., Szabo A., Raglin J., Hettinga F., Roelands B., Lane A., Foad A., Coleman D., and Beedie C., "The Placebo and Nocebo Effect on Sports Performance: A Systematic Review," Eur J Sport Sci (August 2019), https://www.ncbi.nlm.nih.gov/pubmed/31414966.

Likewise, don't be so reliant on a specific routine or circumstance (everything in your schedule "going right") that you're immediately thrown off when something interferes.

Expectations can be used to your detriment or your benefit. Sometimes it's best to not have any expectations at all, and instead deal with what the situation gives you.

What are some of your underlying expectations? Are you inadvertently giving these situations more power than they would otherwise have? How can you better manage your expectations, or at least neutralize them?

Day 85

PLAY WITH WHAT YOU HAVE.

"Each player must accept the cards life deals him or her. But once they are in hand, he or she must decide how to play the cards in order to win the game."
—Voltaire

Today, your cards have been dealt. No one knows what tomorrow will bring and what changes will occur or what challenges you'll face. That's not important anyway.

Today is all you have to influence and change. Regardless of what you're dealing with, how well things may be going, or any unexpected fires you must scramble to smother today, this moment is all there is to work with.

It's easy to think about the way you *wish* things were. "If only the circumstances were different," or "If only this happened at a different time," you say.

But they're not different. Not yet, anyway.

The woman who has neglected self-care for years because she spent every moment caring for her children and family may now find herself overweight and out of shape. "Why did I let this happen?" she may bemoan. The cards are in her hands. All she can do is play with what she has at that moment. The sooner she takes control and plays, the sooner she can move forward.

You can *always* make a move.

The woman who was always active feels discouraged and lost, now that a broken ankle has forced her to take a break from her usual running and strength training routine. She may think she's been dealt a bad hand because she can't run or squat or deadlift; this is a judgment error on her part. There are still *many* moves she can make in this situation, if only she'd stop and see what's there to work with.

Look at what you have to work with. Get creative if you must. You can always make a move. As Theodore Roosevelt said, "Do what you can, with what you have, where you are."

Day 86
CHANGE THE RHETORIC.

For better and worse, social media has greatly affected the way people view working out and moving their bodies.

There's a growing trend of viewing workouts as *going to war* or *preparing for battle,* chanting *sweat is fat crying* and other hyperbolic speech that inflates the significance of moving your body around in space.

It's silly, if not stupid.

Driving to a gym and pushing and pulling weights, regardless of the intensity involved, does not equate to anything heroic, if you really look at what you're doing. Sure, deadlifting three times your bodyweight is an incredible feat of strength. But raising children as a single parent is more impressive. Working a job you don't particularly like to save money for school is impressive. Rescuing an abandoned animal and giving it a loving home is impressive. Speaking up when you see someone being bullied is impressive.

Working out is not a battle or a noble act. Neither is a workout currency ("I *earned* my food!") or penance ("I have to *work off* that dessert") for eating food. Working out in any fashion doesn't make someone a superior being.

Working out is a privilege, a luxury, an enjoyable activity. At best, it's an investment in self-care.

Setting personal records is fun and should be celebrated. But regardless of the goals you want to reap from fitness, view each workout and every bout of physical activity through that lens—that it's a privilege—and see how your mindset evolves.

Day 87
FAST OR SLOW?

There are essentially two ways to go after health and fitness goals.

1. The fast-and-furious approach: Make numerous changes concurrently to produce more noticeable and measurable results in a shorter time period.

2. The slow-and-steady approach: Make small improvements, or create one new habit at a time until it's mastered before making another, using the compounding effect over a larger span of time to produce noticeable results.

Both methods work. The best one for *you* depends on your personality. Some people do best with the fast approach—making numerous changes to their eating and workout habits at once, for example—because seeing results quickly creates motivation to keep going.

Others, however, will become too overwhelmed by the drastic lifestyle overhaul. They may give up soon after starting because the extreme changes were unsustainable and induced stress. They're better off making one change at a time, like focusing exclusively on performing three strength training workouts per week for the first two months. Once they do that consistently, then they can focus on eating a protein- and fiber-rich breakfast every morning or taking lunch to work.

Perhaps you've tried one of those approaches and the results were abysmal. There's a chance the approach wasn't the best one for you, or wasn't the best option at that time.

Keep in mind that just because one approach worked extremely well for a friend, family member, colleague, or social media icon doesn't mean it will work best for *you*. Don't be afraid to blaze your own path. Take the time to figure out what is best for you, right now.

Day 88
THE POWER OF SELF-FULFILLING PROPHECY.

If you repeatedly claim to "suck" at performing a specific skill or task, don't be so surprised when you're right.

"I'm terrible at activities involving cardiorespiratory fitness."

"I can never stick to nutrition changes long term."

"I was born with terrible genes—I'm naturally weak and could never do push-ups."

"I can't learn new skills."

What comments have you made about yourself and your abilities, or lack thereof?

Repeat them enough and they inevitably become your reality.

That is, until you *choose* to do something about it and reforge what is true for you.

The woman who claims to have a weak upper body and proclaims she could never perform a set of push-ups can see this weakness as an opportunity to defeat that preconceived notion. She can follow a program that progresses her push-up strength and shatter that self-imposed limitation.

What could you achieve if you change the stories you tell yourself about your strengths and weaknesses, and create an action-based plan? Instead of self-fulfilling prophecies focusing on your inabilities with negative outcomes, how can you turn them into an advantage or, at the very least, a challenge that will make you mentally, and perhaps even physically, stronger?

Day 89
FRIENDLY REMINDERS.

There are some days when we could all use a helpful reminder. Perhaps one of these will hit the mark for you today:

The number on the scale has no relation to your self-worth.

You do not have to "earn" your food.

You do not have to "work off" any treats either.

Your health and fitness regimen should make you feel great about yourself and, for the most part, be enjoyable.

There's rampant nonsense in the health and fitness industry vying for your attention, and money. They'll attempt to lure you in with promises of "hacks" and shortcuts and secrets. Don't be tempted. Focus your efforts instead on mastering the basics: eating nutrient-dense foods, getting adequate sleep, managing stress, exercising regularly.

You may make less-than-ideal food choices for a day, or a week, or even longer. You can get back to building the habits you want to establish with the next meal.

Every workout will not be great. This is part of fitness. Do what you can, when you can. Don't have an emotional attachment to your workouts.

You don't control many things that happen during the day. You do, however, always have control over your response to them.

Life is too short to waste time obsessing over your eating habits or workout routine or hating parts of your body. Strive to ensure your actions improve your life.

Sometimes the best thing you can do when it comes to health and fitness is to *stop thinking about health and fitness*. It should enhance your life, not dominate it. Go do something else you enjoy.

Day 90

OWN YOUR PERSONAL RECORDS.

Have you ever said something like the following?

"I squatted an all-time personal best today! But I know it's not much weight for others …"

"I did push-ups on the ground for the first time ever; it was just three reps, but I'm pretty happy with it."

"It feels great to press 25-pound dumbbells, but I used to press 40 pounders years ago."

This apologetic tone isn't uncommon, unfortunately. And we need to stop it.

Be proud of your personal records. Embrace your ever-increasing strength, stamina, and abilities. Don't ever allow the "But someone else can do more/better" thoughts or "I used to be able to do more/I should be further along than this" comments hinder your celebration. Don't attach disqualifying words like "just" or "only" or "but" to your accomplishments.

This is *your* journey, and everyone else has their own.

Next time you set a personal record, be proud of yourself. Take note of the achievement and don't allow your eyes to wander to the other women who can lift more/run faster than you. Don't compare where you are now to where you were many years ago or where you feel you "should" be. That doesn't matter.

If anything, look at it this way: You set a personal record or hit a great milestone, and that's awesome. And you likely have more room to get stronger, or faster, or build greater levels of endurance. There are more milestones still yet to be celebrated.

Remember, these milestones can come in many forms: more weight lifted, more reps performed, distance covered in less time, greater resistance used for cardio work; improvements in health markers like blood pressure and cholesterol; habit-building personal bests such as working out consistently each week, enjoying favorite foods guilt free, eating more vegetables each day, not comparing yourself to another person (or a younger version of yourself), and any other action that moves you in the direction you want to go.

Earn your personal records, own them (proudly), and be excited to go do more.

Days 91–100

Day 91
IT WILL NOT BE EASY.

Some people make achieving certain goals—a lean body, world-record crushing levels of strength or endurance, mastering eating habits, embracing a healthy mindset, building a thriving career, intuitive eating—look effortless.

This is especially true on social media and in advertisements. While concealing the truth of their grueling workouts and diet deprivation, some of these sources chant, "It's so easy everyone can do it! What's your excuse?" It seems they never struggle, never miss a step, never have doubts or setbacks.

It doesn't work that way.

You need to not only accept that a healthy lifestyle won't always be easy, especially if you're striving for progressively challenging goals. Instead of asking, "Why is this so hard?" you're better off embracing the fact that challenges are part of the process, and become better at tackling them.

There will be trial and error, ups and downs, highs and lows, personal records and abysmal workouts. The good news is that you can learn from all of it.

The "overnight success" is an illusion, if not an outright lie. Except for the few genetically gifted elite who can achieve dramatic results from even the least amount of strength training (or those who can commit every possible resource to the endeavor), most of us have to put in consecutive months of effort. Many of us will need years to see radical changes to our performance or appearance.

Knowing it will not be easy shouldn't be disappointing or daunting. You just need to correctly manage your expectations of what this journey will look like. You need to see what it will require of you daily, and not be disillusioned by the hype and fabrication spewing from people who think their singular experience is the standard for every other individual.

There is a silver lining: The outcomes we must work the hardest to achieve are often the ones we savor most. It's okay that things aren't always easy. You're not afraid of putting in the work and time.

Day 92

IT'S OKAY TO CHANGE DIRECTION.

When you commit to a certain methodology or program, you probably feel obligated to stick with it. Quitting or choosing a different course of action feels like failure.

However, sometimes changing direction is the better option.

Perhaps you made some nutrition changes to improve your health and boost performance at the gym. But if you're miserable, or it triggers previous unhelpful habits you once defeated, taking a different tack would benefit you.

If your new workout program has you dreading your workouts rather than enjoying them, there's no shame in switching to something you would look forward to. In fact, as you well know by now, enjoyment is an important factor with fitness. You should enjoy what you do, at least most of the time, to ensure you continue doing it.

Likewise, if something you're doing exacerbates old issues, or if your goals just change, it's okay to change direction.

This isn't the same thing as diet hopping out of impatience, or switching a workout program after three weeks because you didn't see drastic changes to your body. You want a sound plan, ideally one you enjoy as much as possible, and you need a hefty combination of consistency and patience.

But if you suspect there's a better way *for you* at any given time, or you have a more motivating goal or focus that necessitates change, boldly adjust course.

Day 93

NOT ABOUT BEING FEARLESS.

"I learned that courage was not the absence of fear, but the triumph over it."

–Nelson Mandela

You want to be courageous enough to do the things that intimidate you. If only you weren't afraid, then you'd be able to get out of your comfort zone and become the person you want to be.

That's incorrect. As Nelson Mandela said, the solution isn't the absence of fear. You simply need to muster up courage to triumph over it.

There's nothing wrong with being intimidated to try something new or face a challenge. The courage to triumph over it is within you. You just may need to coax it out, then hold on tight as it leads you forward.

Sometimes what intimidates you is the very thing you need to run toward and conquer, not retreat from in fear. The moments when you choose to face it and overcome the challenge are when you grow and become more.

Intimidated to enter the weight area of the gym? You just identified your task.

Intimidated to try that activity that interests you? You know what you need to do.

Look at it this way: To build muscle, bone, strength, endurance, action is required. You can't say, "Look at all the wonderful workout equipment I have!" and expect to achieve results just from surrounding yourself with it and looking at it. You must use it, over and over again. Surrounding yourself with the right tools isn't enough; you've got to pick them up and use them.

This is a beautiful reward of strength training—it shows you how strong you can be, and often makes you realize you're stronger than you imagined possible. Grab hold of that empowerment and apply it to other areas of your life.

Forging a more resilient mindset is no different. If you want to be the person that faces obstacles instead of retreats from them, then you must take action. Know things often appear in our minds more difficult than they truly are. The courage you need is within you. It's up to you to utilize it.

To help you take the first step, think about how proud you'll be once you do the very thing that's intimidating you. Then act. As the philosopher Epictetus said thousands of years ago, "First say to yourself what you would be; and then do what you have to do."

Is there something you've wanted to try or do, but haven't because it seems too intimidating or beyond your comfort zone? You've just identified your task.

Day 94

TO WHOM ARE YOU COMPARING YOURSELF?

Do you frequently compare your body to the half-naked "fitness" images paraded on social media?

Do you compare yourself to your friends, coworkers, or siblings?

Do you compare yourself to your favorite social media experts or athletes?

Do you compare who you are today to a younger version of yourself?

What purpose do these comparisons serve? Do they help you in any way? The most likely answer is no. They don't.

You are not the woman on the magazine. You two have very different lives, different genetics, different circumstances, different abilities, different backgrounds. Using her body as a measuring stick for your own is futile.

Likewise, you are in certain ways not who you were 10, 20, or 30 years ago. That woman lived in a different time, with different circumstances. (And the "you" in 10 or 20 years will be different from the "you" of right now.)

You've probably heard the quotation from Theodore Roosevelt, "Comparison is the thief of joy." Maybe it's time to embrace it, and realize comparisons do not help you. When they creep into your mind as you browse social media, thumb through a magazine, or look through old photos, you should reject them. "This isn't helping me, so I'm not going to engage in this."

Being inspired by others and emulating the traits you admire about them is one thing. But comparison is not an accurate measuring stick, so don't use it.

Day 95
PALATE CLEANSE.

If you've been doing the same workout program with the same equipment, exercises, or rep range for months, and your workout motivation is going stale, a palate cleanse could be beneficial.

Do something different for a couple weeks. If you normally train with barbells, switch to dumbbell or even machine-based exercises. If your exercises are usually performed in the 5-10 rep range, perform them in the 12-20 rep range. Strength train three times per week instead of four. Perform exercises as supersets (performing two exercises back-to-back) if you typically use straight sets (performing each exercise on its own before moving on to the next one). Just do something different.

The good thing about a workout palate cleanse is that, unlike your current program, you won't have any impeding expectations to affect your performance. Whereas you may be accustomed to lifting a certain weight with a specific exercise for an exact rep range, changing things up can reignite the joy of training by removing some of these preconceived ideas of what's possible.

The same principle could apply to cardio and other physical activities. If you run, try biking. If you bike, try swimming. If you typically do low-intensity steady-state cardio, try high-intensity intervals.

A change of routine for two to four weeks can be refreshing, mentally and physically. If your workout motivation is going stale, give this a try. If that's not an issue at the moment, keep the workout palate cleanse as an option for the future.

Day 96
QUICKLY GAIN PERSPECTIVE, AGAIN.

You have an expiration date. We all *must* die. Dying is part of the package that comes with life. Regardless of your feelings about this undeniable truth, from the moment you're born, each second moves you closer to your life's inevitable conclusion.

Some people shriek in horror when they ruminate on this reality then immediately shove it out of mind. But it needn't be frightening. In fact, it can provide freedom, if viewed productively. Use the knowledge of the brevity of life to live with a sense of urgency. Do what's important. Spend time with those you cherish. Purge the copious amounts of noise and nonsense that can clutter your life if you don't keep a vigilant watch.

Use this expiration date reminder to help put events and thoughts in perspective once again. Someday, you will be dead. Looking at what you will face today through that lens and letting it soak in, you can already see how a day of less-than-ideal food choices is woefully insignificant. Missing a workout and choosing instead to plop onto the couch after work isn't worth getting upset over. Obsessing over a weight loss goal or strength goal or looking perfect loses its power. You can see how silly it is to allow your happiness to be held hostage by specific weight loss or body-building outcomes.

Put your focus, energy, and limited time where they matter most. And muffle your ears and shield your eyes from the nonsense that attempts to creep in and distract you and blur your vision.

Day 97
REGAIN CONTROL.

Avoidance can be useful. Someone whose day can be ruined from what they see after stepping on the scale in the morning can benefit from avoiding the scale altogether. The person who struggles with portion control and eats a whole sleeve of his favorite cookies instead of the few he planned on can eliminate temptation by not keeping them in the house.

In these two examples, avoidance removes an unhelpful self-judgment and negates the need for willpower, respectively.

But what if you want to regain control and take back the power such situations have over you? You can't simply reintroduce the scenario or food and hope for the best. You must have a plan.

The person who is only happy when the number on the scale goes down, and berates herself if it goes up or stays the same, must first mentally rehearse *what that number means* (objective data only), and do her best to remove the judgment she attaches to it ("I'm a failure if it doesn't go down").

She can acknowledge that the number does not affect her self-worth, that it can be easily manipulated (by water, salt, or carbohydrate intake, for example), that it fluctuates, that it does not provide in-depth information (it doesn't reveal how much muscle and bone she has, her strength or stamina, the habits she's built, etc.). It is just a number revealing the gravitational force between her and Earth. She can *choose* not to add a judgment to it. She can rehearse this each time before, and after, stepping on the scale to gradually eliminate the stigma previously attached to it.

The man who struggles with portion control can divide the package of his favorite cookies into individual servings so he doesn't have to rely on willpower to grab just a couple cookies when he wants to enjoy them. He can remind himself there's no need to feel guilty about eating a favorite food and enjoy a couple cookies daily until the prior anxiety around that food fades.

This is an advanced tactic, so employ it when you're ready. Choose one thing, devise a plan, be diligent, don't demand perfection from the beginning, and you can regain control over something you once relinquished it to.

Day 98
THE MANY COLORS OF SUCCESS.

Success doesn't look the same for everyone. It will look different for different individuals, at different times in their lives.

For one person, success might mean weight loss that leads to improved health measurements.

Success for another might mean gaining weight.

For one person, success might mean not skipping their workouts.

Success for another might mean being able to miss a workout without feeling anxiety or guilt for doing so.

For one person, success might mean eating lean meat, whole grains, and sautéed vegetables for dinner instead of a favorite high-calorie deep-fried meal.

Success for another might mean being able to eat a high-calorie deep-fried meal in a reasonable amount without feeling guilty, like they must "earn" or "work off" the food.

For one person, success might mean practicing self-compassion after a week of less-than-ideal food and fitness choices.

Success for another might mean exercising self-compassion while calling out their own nonsense and objectively seeing where improvement needs to be made.

Don't confuse or compare what means success for *you* with what's pandered on social media (especially since much of it is exaggerated, erroneous, or complete nonsense). This is *your* journey, and it will look different from everyone else's, and can evolve over time.

Day 99
CHANGE IS HARD.

You already know how difficult it can be to establish healthful eating, workout, and self-care habits. To feel like you take two giant steps forward, only to soon after take three backward.

Change is hard.

Building new habits and striving for self-improvement is a challenging endeavor that demands effort and patience. When the realization of this challenge makes itself known, you might revert to the easier way of doing things, the old habits of thought and action.

Here's something that can help you through the difficult times: When you're tempted to quit, or you're discouraged by the effort required of you, pause and think long term.

What will be the long-term outcome of your actions?

Giving up and reverting to old habits will certainly not put you in the place you want to be several months from now. Doing the difficult things *now* will produce positive long-term effects.

Do what you can today and weigh your choices against the future consequences they will produce.

Day 100
PERSEVERE.

How splendid and convenient it would be if we could instantly learn a new skill, overcome a fear, or do something once and have it permanently stamped into our repertoire, making it a reliable habit that doesn't require conscious effort to execute.

That's not how life works, unfortunately. That is why, despite our best efforts to create healthful and helpful habits and demolish unhelpful ones, our journeys are littered with slip-ups, setbacks, obstacles, and even humbling failures.

"I have not failed. I've just found 10,000 ways that won't work," Thomas Edison stated.

We all need to apply that attitude to our health and fitness lifestyle.

You may want nutrition to be easy, to never overthink what you eat, to not obsess about your food choices or to overindulge, to balance saying "no" when necessary with being able to enjoy your favorite foods without guilt. But you won't always get it right. The sooner you know that, and are okay with that fact, the sooner you too can say, "I haven't failed; I've just found what doesn't work for me." Acknowledge it and keep going, or else start from scratch and construct a fresh plan.

To quote Thomas Edison once more, "Our greatest weakness lies in giving up. The most certain way to succeed is always to try just one more time."

Perseverance must become your motto. Know that obstacles and setbacks are inevitable; expecting their arrival will take away their sting. Face them as best you can by embracing the strength and stamina you've built throughout this journey, extract any possible lessons from them, then continue on your path. Try one more time.

There's a Latin phrase that perfectly expresses this: *vires acquirit eundo*—"we gather strength as we go."

Some things we can learn or change quickly. Others will take much more time and effort. Your journey *begins* here. Keep practicing. Keep taking action. Keep learning. Keep persevering.

Conclusion
NOW WHAT?

Just because you've reached the end of this book does not mean your journey has concluded. Really, the exact opposite has happened. You're beginning a *new* chapter.

Depending on where you started, you may still have work to do in certain areas of your health and fitness lifestyle. That's not just okay; it's to be expected. Be proud of the progress you've made to this point and continue to put in the effort to improve where desired. You'll make quicker progress in certain areas, and in others you'll need greater patience and persistence.

Whatever you do, don't stop now. Keep going.

ABOUT THE AUTHOR

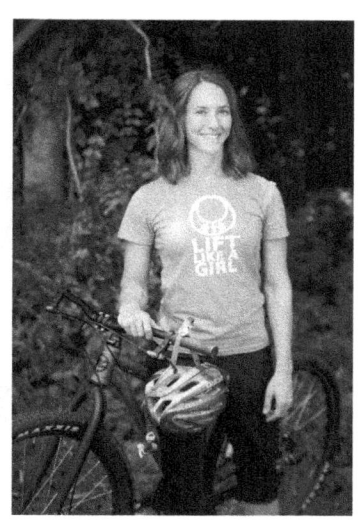

Nia Shanks is a fitness coach and writer with a bachelor of science in exercise physiology from the University of Louisville. She specializes in helping women "be more!" with an empowering approach to health and fitness. Nia's philosophy revolves around strength training programs with a focus on getting stronger and helping women discover the incredible things their bodies can do, and she promotes obsession-free, flexible nutrition principles. Through her popular blog and online coaching courses, Nia has helped thousands of women look beyond "quick weight loss" and discover the amazing body they never knew they had.

www.NiaShanks.com

Also by Nia Shanks

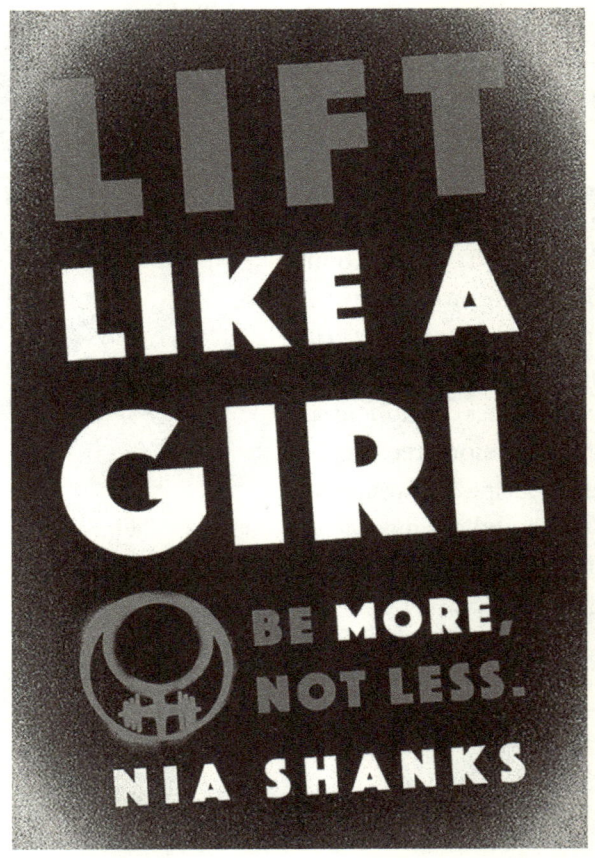

www.ingramcontent.com/pod-product-compliance
Lightning Source LLC
LaVergne TN
LVHW090309191224
799449LV00003B/241